SO-BSY-909

"Bravo Dr. Rivas, finally an excellent, refreshing look at obesity and a novel approach to its treatment for those of us in the trenches fighting what previously was a losing battle. This is a must read for anyone concerned with treating obesity of suffering with it!"

RALPH J. LA GUARDIA M.D.

"Paul Rivas, M.D. is the vanguard for the current and future treatment of obese patients. His sections regarding treatment are well thought out and easy to understand. His remark regarding some doctors who blame the patient for being overweight are sadly too true. Very few American doctors are well trained in the treatment of obesity. Patients and doctors, read this, please!"

A. RANDALL MOSS, M.D.
Gaffney Family Physicians, Carolina Slender Center

"I've used the advice given in this book myself and with my patients with extraordinary success. Dr. Rivas is the master of weight control."

ROBERT STOLTZ, M.D.
Internal Medicine
(and a patient of Dr. Rivas's)

"I've seen first-hand hundreds of patients who have achieved and maintained incredible weight losses through Dr. Rivas when absolutely nothing else worked. The guy's a genius."

TAMMY DRESSEL, R.N.
Baltimore, Maryland

"When the pills are working, it's like night and day. The schedule, the stress, the environment—nothing matters! It's easy."

CHERYL COGAR, R.N.

TURN OFF THE
HUNGER
Switch

RESET YOUR BRAIN TO CHANGE YOUR WEIGHT

PAUL RIVAS, M.D.

FOREWORD BY RICHARD ROTHMAN, M.D.,Ph.D.

PRENTICE HALL

Library of Congress Cataloging-in-Publication Data

Rivas, Paul.
    Turn off the hunger switch / by Paul Rivas.
       p. cm.
    Includes index.
    ISBN 0-13-060563-8 — ISBN 0-7352-0300-8
    1. entry.   2. entry.   3. entry.   4. entry.   I. Title.

    RM222.2 .R553 2001
    613.7—dc21   2001036787

Acquisitions Editor: *Ernie Tremblay*
Production Editor: *Eve Mossman*
Page Design/Layout: *Robyn Beckerman*

©2002 by Paul Rivas

All rights reserved. No part of this book may be reproduced in any form or by any means, without permission in writing from the publisher.

Printed in the United States of America

10 9 8 7 6 5 4 3 2 1

This publication contains the opinions and ideas of its author and is designed to provide useful advice in regard to the subject matter covered. The author and publisher are not engaged in rendering medical or other professional services in this publication. This publication is not intended to provide a basis for action in particular circumstances without consideration by a competent health professional. The author and publisher expressly disclaim any responsibility for any liability, loss, or risk, personal or otherwise, which is incurred as a consequence, directly or indirectly, of the use and application of any of the contents of this book.

ISBN 0-13-060563-8

ATTENTION: CORPORATIONS AND SCHOOLS

Prentice Hall books are available at quantity discounts with bulk purchase for educational, business, or sales promotional use. For information, please write to: Prentice Hall Special Sales, 240 Frisch Court, Paramus, New Jersey 07652. Please supply: title of book, ISBN, quantity, how the book will be used, date needed.

PRENTICE HALL
Paramus, NJ 07652

http://www.phdirect.com

Obesity is a serious medical condition. Before beginning any weight loss program, you should consult with a licensed health care provider. This book is intended as a source of information and reference volume only, not as a medical guide. The information provided is intended to help the reader make informed decisions about his or her health, but is in no way intended as a substitute for the personal care of a physician and professional medical treatment. Likewise, weight loss medications and supplements may have significant physiological effects and side effects, and should be taken only under the supervision of a qualified professional, to whom you should report all side effects you experience. In particular, prescription medicines such as those discussed throughout this book should never be obtained or taken except in consultation with a physician. Chapter 9 and Appendix C of this book are intended to assist you in finding the right medical professional for your particular weight loss needs, and you are urged to make use of these resources and consult with a licensed health care provider before embarking on any weight loss program.

Contents

Foreword

Doctors call the state of being overweight obesity. Over 58 million people in the United States fall into that category, and the numbers are increasing.

The health risks of obesity are well documented. As noted in an editorial in the *New England Journal of Medicine* (vol. 335, pp. 659–660, 1996), "Obesity is the second leading cause of preventable death in the United States exceeded only by cigarette smoking." Obesity is a major risk factor for cardiovascular illnesses such as hypertension, elevated blood cholesterol, and coronary artery disease. Obesity is also a major risk factor for developing diabetes and certain cancers.

Many informed members of the public already know these facts. Less well appreciated is the strong association of obesity with the development of low back pain, joint pain, and fractures of the hip, especially in the elderly, and, as reported in a 1995 study published in the *New England Journal of Medicine*, even modest degrees of obesity increases the risk of premature death.

The benefits of weight reduction are documented by careful medical research. Blood cholesterol comes down, blood pressure begins to normalize, and blood sugar improves with even small amounts of weight loss.

Many people, including health professionals, think of obesity as being a "willpower" disease. These people believe that if overweight individuals would only control their appetites, then they would most certainly reverse their weight problems. The fact that many obese patients cannot, despite great effort, control their appetites, or do not lose weight even when they do, is taken as evidence that obese individuals lack the willpower possessed by thinner people. This conceptualization of obesity, which blames the victim of a disease for having the disease, is not supported by scientific and medical research. In fact, it's simply wrong.

Traditional approaches to weight reduction include a changed diet, increased aerobic exercise, and behavioral modification. Unfortunately, they just don't work for many patients, and over long periods of time, they seem to work for very few. For these patients, treatment with anorectic agents (substances that can help you lose or control your weight) can be helpful.

In this book, Paul Rivas, M.D., delves into this complex area with expertise and astute insight. Building on his extensive clinical experience in treating obesity, his acute clinical acumen, and his broad knowledge of the medical literature, Dr. Rivas makes this complex subject understandable to the lay person. He provides useful examples and helpful advice for people trying to lose weight.

I highly recommend this book not only to people embarking on a weight-loss program, but also to anyone who seeks a deeper understanding of obesity, its causes, and its treatments.

Richard B. Rothman, M.D., Ph.D.

Introduction

I am a bariatrician, a doctor who treats people who find it difficult to control their weight—and today, I am a *successful* bariatrician. My patients actually lose weight and keep it off. But it hasn't always been so.

Like most weight-loss doctors, when I first began my practice, I immediately ran up against a brick wall. I had gone through standard medical training at a good medical school, so I offered everyone who came to see me the standard medical advice I had learned: Eat less and exercise more. The problem was that my advice didn't work. Most of my patients weren't getting any thinner, and those who were didn't stay that way for long.

Then one patient, Roy M., came in one day and did something that would forever change the way I practiced medicine.

Roy had been coming to my office for years, desperately looking for a way to control his weight, but he just couldn't seem to make any progress. The problem was that he loved Italian food, craved it so much, in fact, that he felt completely helpless to resist when in the presence of a beckoning bowl of pasta. Finally, at my wits' end, I accused him of being a bad patient. He didn't bother to point out my failure as a doctor. He simply asked me for pills to control his appetite.

If you have ever gone to your family physician, or even a bariatrician, and asked for diet pills, you already know this story. Pills are precisely what you do not get. What you probably do get is a stern look (or if you're lucky, a benevolent one) and a pamphlet that tells you to count your calories, cut down your fat intake, and do more exercise. What you probably also get is the feeling that your doctor does not take your problem seriously. You are not like his or her other patients, patients who are genuinely sick.

So it was with Roy. I told him I did not believe in diet pills and had never prescribed them in ten years of practice.

Why not?

Until recently, most diet medications came from the amphetamine family. These drugs are powerful appetite inhibitors, but they are also dangerous and addicting. People who use them over an extended period of time often become restless and nervous. Many develop the "shakes," a chronic and noticeable trembling of the hands. Insomnia is common. Overdoses can cause depression, psychosis, and death. These were not drugs I would give to people I care about—and I care very much about my patients. I didn't realize at the time that science was already discovering new tools—many of them natural supplements as powerful as medications—in the fight against obesity.

As for Roy, I was convinced that, for some odd reason, he was choosing ravioli over self-esteem and good health. Losing weight, I thought, was simply a matter of making better choices and keeping one's self under better control. Not such a difficult thing for a person to do. After all, I controlled my eating habits, didn't I? Surely his temptations were no worse than mine.

Or were they?

Finally frustrated and out of patience, Roy handed me a copy of a report by Dr. Michael Weintraub. That moment was the beginning of a revolution in my thinking that has changed Roy's life, those of my patients, and perhaps most of all, my own.

In my years of practice since then, I've treated nearly 12,000 patients for their overweight condition, with close to a 95-percent success rate. All of those patients have driven home one fact for me that may contradict everything you have ever heard on the subject: Dieting and exercise have nothing to do with weight loss.

I know it sounds unlikely. I know it goes against common sense. But it's true. Don't take my word for it. Just look at the world around you.

Diet books are perennial bestsellers, even though they very often contradict one another. One proposes high carbohydrates; another, high proteins; still another, high fats. Some claim that simply balancing your meals will do the trick. Others suggest changing your eating habits according to your blood type or the season of the year. In the meantime, we spend millions of dollars on treadmills, tummy-toning exercise machines, and health-club memberships.

Unfortunately, despite all this effort, we don't seem to be losing any weight. Nearly everyone who loses weight through diet and exercise gains it back within five years.

In my own practice, patients often come to me in utter confusion and despair after years of exhausting exercising and restricted eating with little or no weight loss to show for it. In fact, many have watched in horror as the needle on the scale actually moved *upward* when they cut their calories back. They feel weak and out of control.

"What's wrong with me?" they'll say. "What diet should I be on and how much should I exercise?" Or "Maybe I should just give up and accept myself as I am."

My answer is usually not what they expect to hear. In fact, it's something that most people have never heard before: The sizes of your meals don't matter, but the size of your appetite does. It's not the degree to which you consume food, but the degree to which you crave and desire food that controls your weight. It's not so much the steaks, chocolate, and fries, but rather the obsessions with them that ultimately add fat to your frame.

Why? Insatiable hunger tells your body to go into its fat-storing mode. Your system feels the symptoms of starvation, so it stops "wasting" precious calories by burning them and stockpiles them instead.

So, I tell my patients, don't worry about eating that piece of chocolate, but rather how much you crave it.

What controls how much you crave and obsess over food? It has nothing to do with your diet; it has to do with your parents. It's not your exercise program that matters; it's your genetic program. The solution to your problem doesn't lie in willpower, self-control, or pushing away from the table. It lies turning off your appetite, and your appetite center is located in your brain.

Once you do that, chocolate and sweets will instantly lose their appeal. You'll feel full after eating only a small portion of a meal. Food thoughts and compulsive eating stop. It's instant, dramatic, and works exceptionally well.

So put away your weight-loss books, throw away your tummy toners, and learn how to turn off your hunger switch. The day of the diet is over.

Paul Rivas, M.D.

1

Hard Facts About Soft Tissue

Fat is unhealthy. You already know this. You see it on television, hear it on the radio, and read it in books, magazines,
and newspapers. Every lethal disease you can think of seems
to have some connection with eating red meat, dairy products, sauces, and pastries. Responsible health organizations
the world over recommend a diet high in fruits, grains, and
vegetables, and low in beef, milk, butter, and eggs.

The warning is clear: Putting too much fat into your
stomach will make you sick—but so will putting too much fat
around your stomach.

How much is too much? When we glance at the mirror,
most of us don't see a problem. We may be sporting "love
handles" or even a little "mid-life paunch," but that, we tell
ourselves, doesn't make us dangerously heavy. Obese people

1

Are You in the Danger Zone?

If you're carrying excess pounds, your health is in serious jeopardy. Too much fat can kill you.

How much is too much?

Until recently, doctors made that determination by looking at your body weight. Now there is a much more powerful tool for recognizing obesity. It's called the *body mass index* or BMI. To determine your BMI, you have to do a little arithmetic. Multiply your weight in pounds by 705. Divide that number by your height in inches. Then divide your answer by your height in inches again.

Weight x 705 ÷ Height in inches ÷ Height in inches = BMI

You can use this chart for to find your BMI quickly:

BMI

Weight	Height					
	5'0"	5'3"	5'6"	5'9"	6'0"	6'3"
140 lbs	27	25	23	21	19	18
150 lbs	29	27	24	22	20	19
160 lbs	31	28	26	24	22	20
170 lbs	33	30	28	25	23	21
180 lbs	35	32	29	27	25	23
190 lbs	37	34	31	28	26	24
200 lbs	39	36	32	30	27	25
210 lbs	41	37	34	31	29	26
220 lbs	43	39	36	33	30	28
230 lbs	45	41	37	34	31	29
240 lbs	47	43	39	36	33	30
250 lbs	49	44	40	37	34	31

If your BMI falls within the range of 25 to 27, you're moderately overweight; from 27 to 30, you're obese; and over 30, you're seriously obese.

are more like those fat ladies in the circus. They look like Mama Cass Eliot or John Candy. *Those* are the people who die from being overweight.

Bariatricians will tell you otherwise. They've seen the numbers. They know that many people who call themselves "pleasingly plump" or "a little overweight" can fall well within the danger zone of obesity—and that is a very dangerous place indeed.

THE PRICE TO YOUR HEALTH

If *you* fall within that zone, you are at greater risk for diabetes, heart disease, blood vessel disease, gallbladder disease, arthritis, and high blood pressure. You're also more likely to get cancer of the colon.

If you're an overweight male, your chances of developing prostate cancer are higher. If you're a plus-size female, you need to be more concerned about cancers of the ovaries and uterus than thin women do.

There is one glimmer of good news for overweight women: You're less at risk for heart disease than are your male counterparts—so long as you bear most of your extra weight below your waist, rather than around it. But your risk for breast cancer rises to one and a half times the average.

The picture becomes even more complicated—and frightening—if you're obese and pregnant. Your odds for bearing a baby with a debilitating birth defect double if you're seriously overweight (BMI [body mass index] of 27–30) and quadruple if you're dangerously obese (BMI over 30). The two most common of these defects are spina bifida, which can paralyze a child, and anencephaly, a condition in which most of the brain is missing.

For some reason researchers don't yet understand, folic acid supplements reduce the risk of these defects in child-bearing women of normal weight, but have no effect whatsoever when taken by overweight mothers-to-be.

THE SOCIAL COST

Statistics concerning your health become worse and worse as your weight goes up, but health isn't the only issue. People who are noticeably overweight also have to contend with prejudice, rejection, and scorn.

It's sad but true: If you suspect you were passed over for a promotion, denied a job, or simply not invited to a party because of your size, you're probably right.

According to studies, a majority of college students claim they would rather marry a drug dealer or a thief than an obese person. Six-year-old children commonly call fat kids "dirty," "cheats," "liars," "ugly," and "stupid." Most surprising of all, even doctors often describe overweight patients as "weak-willed, ugly, and awkward."

What are you supposed to do about all this? Some people simply decide to be proud of who they are, no matter how heavy they may be. They make a conscious decision not to lose weight. That's praiseworthy—to a point—but it addresses only the issue of self-esteem, not health. Whatever you've heard in the news about being overweight *and* physically fit, exercise will improve only your circulatory and heart health. Your risk for cancer, diabetes, and arthritis remain dangerously high.

For most us, there can be only one decision: Take control of our lives and our health by losing weight.

Simple.

SIMPLE? ARE YOU OUT OF YOUR MIND?

"If losing weight is so simple, why does every approach I try work wonderfully for about five minutes before I start putting the pounds back on again?"

Good question. In fact, chances are good that there's not a weight-loss plan or product on the market you haven't tested on yourself with lousy results. You've been through the struggle of trying to resist overwhelming cravings. You've starved yourself week after week, only to end up on the food binge of all food binges. You've forced yourself to jog, stair climb, and aerobicize until you have the stamina of a cross-country runner. You've swallowed enough "fat burners" to melt all the candles in the Vatican.

Worst of all, after turning your life into a boot camp and finally losing some weight, you've watched in horror as those lost pounds reappeared out of nowhere and attached themselves again, like stalkers waiting in ambush.

Now, you hardly put a crumb to your mouth, let alone overeat, yet you seem to get bigger and bigger. Imagining an entire lifetime on this merry-go-round is depressing to say the least.

To make matters even worse, we see people all around us who seem to maintain a healthy weight and slender body with no effort whatsoever. They're the same people who criticize us for not controlling calorie intake. They eat what they want, when they want, and in whatever amount they want, but they never gain a pound. They look like a bunch of long-distance runners, though we know for a fact that many of them are couch potatoes. Exercise doesn't seem to make any difference.

What's going on here? Is there some fundamental, underlying physical difference between thin people and fat people? Science tells us there is.

CHIPS OFF THE OLD BLOCK

In 1988, the *New England Journal of Medicine* published the results of a Danish study of 540 people who had been adopted during infancy. The subjects of the study were divided into four groups: thin, normal weight, overweight, and obese. Their weights were then compared with those of their adopted parents and their biological parents. You might expect that the adoptees would mostly end up in the same weight class as that of their adoptive parents. After all, people in the same home would eat the same foods at the same mealtimes, and probably in similar quantities. The results, however, pointed in the other direction. Adoptees had a much stronger tendency to end up in the weight class of their *biological* parents.

Other research has yielded similar results. A 1986 study, published in the *Journal of the American Medical Association,* compared the weights of both adult identical twins and fraternal twins. If genetics were the important factor in body mass, then identical twins should grow up to be in the same weight class—and that's exactly what happened. The authors, using three different methods of analyzing their data, came to the conclusion that ". . . human fatness is under strong genetic control."

More recently, researchers have learned some of the ways in which genetics exert that control. At the University of California, scientists have discovered a gene that determines whether the fat you consume will burn off as harmless body heat or go into storage as adipose. In Great Britain, another team of investigators has found a protein, GLP-1, that signals the brain when you've had enough to eat. Similarly, the hormone leptin may be at least partially responsible for maintaining body weight at an unmoving level.

The Role of Metabolism

"My metabolism is slow." Doctors hear it all the time from overweight patients. "If I eat any less, I'll die of starvation, but I still can't seem to lose a pound." This is usually the point at which the doctor's eyes will glaze over. The doctor may be nodding his or her head in sympathy, but the doctor is actually thinking, "She's deluding herself and making excuses. The less you eat, the more weight you lose. If you're not losing, then you're eating too much. End of story." Meanwhile, the patient is thinking, "My body just doesn't burn calories the way other people's do. If I'm fat, it's because I have a built-in handicap."

Who's right? Probably neither. When a person has a low metabolic rate relative to his or her size, studies show that the person is also more likely to be carrying around too much body weight. The Pima Indians, who have, on average, slower metabolisms than nearly any other group of people in the world, also have the highest prevalence of obesity. But there is no clear evidence that a slow metabolism and obesity are related by cause and effect, only that the two conditions occur in the same people. There is much stronger evidence that they're both effects of a more fundamental cause: a genetic predisposition.

One of the most interesting and peculiar effects of genetics on body weight is a strong inherited tendency to like or dislike certain foods. Scientists announced this finding a few years ago at a meeting of the American Association for the Advancement of Science. Apparently, people divide broadly into three groups: super-tasters, tasters, and non-tasters. Because they've inherited more taste buds, super-tasters actually taste more of the bitterness and sweetness in what they eat than do others. Non-tasters can put virtually anything in their mouths to little or no effect. Naturally, the amounts and kinds of foods each group tends to consume are vastly different.

Heredity is so firmly connected to the problem of being overweight that 80 percent of the offspring of two overweight parents will become obese, as compared with only 14 percent of two parents who are of normal weight. But if heredity is so important, why do Japanese people still living in Japan generally remain thin, while their counterparts who have moved to the West become as fat as Europeans and Americans?

Heredity may create strong tendencies, but environment creates opportunities. Who knows how many Heifitzes and Perlmans lived and died before the invention of the violin? No matter how great the talent, if there is no fiddle, there is no fiddler. Likewise with obesity. In cultures where high-calorie foods are hard to come by, such as Japan and China, potentially overweight people remain thin. In the West, however, there is ample opportunity to eat fats, sugars, and starches, and we take advantage of it.

SITUATION HOPEFUL

Luckily for us, science is not all grim news. Bad genes don't make obesity inevitable, and we're beginning to understand the mechanism by which they do their dirty work.

If you give it some thought, you can probably pinpoint the specific time in your life when you began gaining weight.

Perhaps it happened after some particularly stressful event, such as taking a new medicine and/or hormonal therapy; going through surgery, pregnancy, or a divorce; or suffering the loss of a loved one through death. Or it could have occurred simply as a result of reaching a certain age. You may have gotten heavy when you were young, or you may have been thin for the first several decades of your life before your weight suddenly spiraled out of control—despite the lack of any significant change in exercise or eating habits. As many overweight people say, it's as if a fat-storing switch had been turned on inside your body.

What a frustrating experience, to see your weight climbing and climbing, to find yourself obsessing over food all day every day, and to feel so completely powerless to stop the process! Yet it was exactly this situation that gave us the clues we needed to solve the mystery of obesity and the answers we needed to bring you the most life-altering news you'll ever hear:

There is a "fat-storing switch" in the body that can suddenly, and without warning, flip to the "on" position. But if you know how, *you can just as suddenly turn it off again!*

2

Hunting the Elusive Fat-Storing Switch

In order to flip the switch, you first have to know where to find it, and therein lies the problem. For a very long time, we've been looking in all the wrong places.

A CHARACTER FLAW?

The first place we tried was that hard-to-pin-down quality of the human personality we call "character." We didn't look very closely at the conclusions we leapt to because we believed they were self-evident. Here was the logic: Whenever you eat, any energy you don't immediately burn you store as fat. The more you eat, the more you put into storage and the fatter you become. Since many people manage to control their eating habits and remain at a healthy weight, people who don't obviously lack self-control. In other words, they have a *character flaw.*

The problem with this reasoning is obvious. Many, if not most, overweight people have spent much of their lives depriving themselves of food—often surviving on a ridiculously low intake of calories—despite experiencing very poor results in keeping off the pounds. What could show more self-discipline? They bring this same determination to exercise. When it comes to strength of character, many thin people could take a lesson from their heavier brothers and sisters.

NEXT STOP, THE MIND

All right, then, if the problem wasn't a character flaw, then perhaps it was subtler in nature. If the typical overweight person often deprived him- or herself of food, it was still true that the person's behavior—frequently bingeing or chronically overeating—seemed to bring about his or her weight woes. So what was causing the behavior, some *psychological* problem?

When doctors tell their patients that losing weight is primarily a psychological problem, what are they really saying?

The theory goes something like this: eating too much is a nervous response, a way to distract yourself from feeling uncomfortable. Any discomfort—including stress, depression, fatigue, anxiety, premenstrual syndrome, shyness, force of habit, or a hundred other situations—can trigger a food binge. So if you want to stop yourself from overeating, you simply need to find other ways of dealing with your discomfort. Bite your nails, blow your top, take up a hobby, or jog a few miles. But whatever else you do, learn to keep your mouth shut in the presence of food.

In other words, it was the same old "character flaw" argument, dressed up in slightly fancier clothing.

COULD 12-STEP PROGRAMS BE THE ANSWER?

If the problem wasn't in the character and it wasn't in the mind, then perhaps we were looking in the wrong direction. Maybe the problem was actually in the *food.*

This reasoning led us to some pretty odd suspicions, the first of which was that food might be an addictive substance for some people. Some researchers even cited evidence for "withdrawal symptoms," which food addicts might experience if they didn't consume their addicting substance.

The addiction theory is a step up from the old way of thinking about obesity, in that it no longer victimizes the victims; that is, it no longer points an accusing finger at overweight people to blame them for their problem. But on closer inspection, it doesn't make much sense.

Any addicting substance hooks its prey by means of some chemical property in the substance itself. Alcohol, tobacco, and cocaine all produce biochemical changes in the human body that, among other symptoms, cause the body to need more of the addicting substance just to keep performing normal activities. Many drugs reinforce the addiction with a sense of euphoria. If you don't take the substance, you can't function; but if you do take the substance, you feel absolutely wonderful! The addiction turns insidious. The more you take, the more you need. This is called tolerance.

Food presents a different picture. We all need it to survive, but no one needs it more than anyone else. There is nothing in the food itself that addicts people to it. It doesn't produce real euphoria, and reports of "withdrawal symptoms" are at best questionable.

As for increased tolerance, if obese people were truly addicted, we would see them eating bigger and bigger meals day by day. Study after study shows that this just doesn't happen.

NOT ADDICTION, BUT OBSESSION

Here is where the story gets interesting. Overweight people may not eat more food, but they sure do think more about it! Most are constantly preoccupied with the subject, even right after eating a large meal. They know their stomachs are full, but somehow they don't feel satisfied.

They think about food when they wake up in the morning, they think about it all through the day, and they think about it when they go to bed in the evening. Sometimes they even wake up in the middle of the night thinking about it! They crave, they binge, they pick, they nibble. And its true: They sometimes eat when they're bored, anxious, stressed, irritable, or angry.

But they also eat when they're relaxed and feeling good.

This is a portrait of neither a weak-willed person nor a typical addict. It is, however, very much like a picture of another class of patients: people with obsessive–compulsive disorder, or OCD. We've all heard about this disease. It leads to irrational, even ritualistic patterns of behavior, over which the victim seems to have no control. An obsession with cleanliness that leads to compulsive hand washing is typical: People will wash their hands to the point of scrubbing off layers of skin, even though they know that what they're doing makes no sense and that it's hurting them. They just can't help themselves.

The similarity between OCD and food obsession suggested that we look for the hunger switch in another location altogether: the chemistry of the brain.

People with OCD have an underlying biochemical abnormality, which may involve the brain substance called serotonin. While we are not yet completely sure that a lack of sufficient serotonin in the brain lies at the bottom of this problem, we do know that serotonin reuptake inhibitors, such as Prozac®, Paxil®, and Zoloft®, help these patients enormously. Not only do patients stop their irrational behavior, but they stop obsessing as well.

Could obesity be treated in a similar way?

GROUND ZERO: THE HUNGER SWITCH

Appetite and weight control begin in a sort of control center of the brain called the hypothalamus. One of the "switchboards" in the center, known as the *ventromedial region,* is in charge of telling you when you've had enough to eat; that is, it's the place that sends you the signal that you're full. If this part of the brain is somehow badly damaged, enormous hunger and obesity always result. A laboratory rat will actually eat itself to death when its ventromedial region is destroyed.

The feeling of hunger comes from yet another control center, the *lateral hypothalamus.* If this area is damaged, loss of appetite and extreme thinness result.

By increasing brain levels of certain substances (including serotonin) that act as triggers for these two controllers in the hypothalamus, not only can we suppress appetite and overeating, but we can also liberate people from obsessing over food!

15

A Direct Approach: Brain Surgery

It's an old, accepted piece of wisdom that, when solving patients' medical problems, internists like to give medicine and surgeons like to operate. It should come as no surprise, then, that a new way to flip the hunger switch was presented at the 49th Annual Meeting of the Congress of Neurological Surgeons: brain surgery.

David A. Vincent, M.D., presented his experimental findings after using a "Gamma" knife (a machine that focuses several beams of gamma radiation on one point in the brain without opening up the skull) to irradiate the hypothalamuses of 36 subjects. Follow-up observations ran for 34 weeks. The results of the experiment demonstrated that the "weight thermostats" of the subjects had been lowered to a healthy level, they all lost weight, and there were no adverse side effects. Only one problem: The subjects, in this case, were lab rats.

No, we're not quite ready to perform brain surgery as a weight-loss remedy for humans. But the study clearly demonstrated one thing: There is a thermostat in the brain that can turn off the hunger switch. It was great news for everyone concerned with helping people to lose weight. Fortunately, irradiating the brain is not the only option.Suppose, however, that you don't really obsess over food. You don't spend all your time thinking about it, but now and again, maybe late at night, just before bed, you have a tremendous craving for something sugary or full of fat. It's interesting that the brain doesn't target vegetables or whole-grain foods when it springs one of these compulsions on you. It goes right for the unhealthiest thing on the menu, and perhaps with good reason.

Dr. Richard Wurtman, Director of the Clinical Research Center at MIT, contends that the brain is actually medicating itself: "We observe that a sizable portion of obese subjects seeking assistance in weight reduction consume as much as half of their total daily intake as carbohydrate-rich snacks, and that the behavior is often associated with strong feelings of carbohydrate cravings. Conceivably, this appetite disorder reflects an abnormality in the process that couples carbohydrate consumption to the release of brain serotonin. Many patients describe themselves as feeling anxious, tense, or depressed before consuming the carbohydrate snack and peaceful or relaxed afterward. . . . Perhaps the subjects snacking on carbohydrate are unknowingly self-medicating."

In other words, they're trying to flip that switch.

FROM BAD GENES TO PLUS SIZE

Since the tendency toward being overweight is clearly inherited, it's a good bet that these "bad genes" do most of their dirty work by causing imbalances in brain chemistry. In turn, these imbalances cause excessive hunger or the inability to get full, cravings for salty or sweet foods, and compulsive eating even when you're not hungry.

But the story doesn't end there. When any of these symptoms appear, the brain signals the body to go into a starvation–storage mode. That means you become extremely efficient at using energy, leaving you able to store, as fat, almost everything you eat, and unable to breakdown any fat you've stored previously.

That's why so many overweight people complain that they're eating like birds and still not losing weight. It also

....

The Gene with a Double Whammy

It's bad enough that a gene could predispose us toward obesity, but it turns out that one such "fat" gene, called HMG I-C, is even worse: It also predisposes us toward cancer.

According to a laboratory study published in the May 2000 issue of *The Journal of Biological Chemistry*, HMG I-C may cause benign tumors, called lipomas, to grow in fat tissue. In themselves, these tumors are harmless, but as they grow, many turn into a type of cancer called malignant liposarcoma.

The good news is that these tumors grow only in fat tissue—so now we have one more reason to keep body fat to a minimum.

....

explains why a thin person, whose brain chemicals are in balance and whose internal engine burns fat faster than a race car burns gasoline, can eat whatever he or she wants and remain thin.

The mechanism works like a thermostat. When your genetic blueprint tilts your brain chemistry out of balance, the "fat-storing thermostat" in the hypothalamus rises to a high setting, and your body will do whatever it takes to reach the weight that setting demands. As you reach the setting, weight gain stops; people do not gain indefinitely. They hover within a few pounds around the set point.

If all this is true, then why aren't fat people born fat? How is it they can often pinpoint the time in their life when they gained much of their weight? Although imbalances in brain chemistry may be genetically determined, it often takes a trigger to set them off. These include stressful life events, like those mentioned in the previous chapter. Unfortunately, simply getting rid of the trigger does not reverse the process.

We had finally found the switch, nestled deep in the human brain. Now we had to figure out a way to turn it off.

3

From Switch
to Switchboard

Back in the early 1990s, we thought we'd found the answer in a combination of two new appetite suppressants—phentermine and fenfluramine.

Phentermine is part of a drug family known as the *central adrenergics*. Phentermine increases the amount of two substances, norepinephrine and dopamine, in the brain. These, in turn, suppress appetite.

Fenfluramine causes cells to release another neurotransmitter, serotonin, directly into the brain, which also suppresses appetite. But serotonin performs a couple of other neat tricks as well: It lifts your mood and it gets rid of cravings, especially for carbohydrates.

The Snack Effect

Most overweight people actually eat about the same number of calories per day as their normal-weight counterparts, but they consume far more of those calories as starchy or sweet snacks. Why? Carbohydrates alter your mood by raising the level of serotonin in the brain. When that happens, all your worries seem to fly away. Serotonin does the same thing—without the added calories.

Dr. Judith Wurtman of the Department of Nutrition at MIT dramatically demonstrated this effect in a field study. She divided her subjects into two groups. People in the first group were given fenfluramine. Those in the second, the control group, were given placebos. The placebo takers ate, on average, five to six snacks per day. Patients using the medication, however, reduced their snack intake by 41 percent, without reducing their consumption of healthy foods at all. In other words, fenfluramine had selectively eliminated their desire to snack!

THE NUMBERS LOOKED GOOD

How did we know all this? How did we know that the drugs would actually work the way they were supposed to and help people to lose weight?

Preliminary studies had already been done on the medications in the late 1970s. Then, in 1989, the results of the first major study appeared in a highly respected British medical journal, *The Lancet.*

Research scientists had carried out a one-year-long experiment using the drug dexfenfluramine (a close relative of fenfluramine), along with a calorie-restricted diet, on 822 overweight patients living all over Europe. The researchers wanted to know if obesity, which they called a "chronic, harmful disorder," could be safely treated with drugs on a long-term basis. After all, they reasoned, you could control chronic diabetes, high blood pressure, and high triglycerides with medication, so why not one of the chief underlying causes of these conditions?

The results were promising. At the end of the study, the European patients had enjoyed significant weight loss—over 10 percent of their starting weight—with only minor, transient side effects.

Then, in 1992, Dr. Michael Weintraub and a team of scientists at the University of Rochester concluded a four-year study of phentermine and fenfluramine. Used together in low doses, the drugs helped over a hundred patients lose an average of almost 16 percent of their body weight in about eight months (against a 4.6-percent average weight loss in a control group). That meant that a 200-pound patient taking these medications would have lost about 32 pounds!

The following year, one of the world's most respected obesity researchers, Dr. Richard Atkinson, at the University of Wisconsin, reported the results of a study he had made.

Atkinson had been giving phentermine and fenfluramine to a group of patients consisting of 57 men and 506 women, and he had presented his findings at the annual meeting of the North American Association for the Study of Obesity. The Associated Press picked up the story.

After three months, his patients had lost an average of 22 pounds. After six months, the average jumped to 29 pounds, and after nine months, 37 pounds!

THE NEWS GETS BETTER

Weight loss was only part of the story. In 49 of the patients in Atkinson's study, blood pressure dropped to normal, while 24 patients saw their cholesterol levels plummet. There was even some evidence that blood sugar had normalized in several diabetic patients. "Dramatic stuff!" was the way Atkinson put it in an article in the *Baltimore Sun* in 1993.

A workshop conducted at the National Institutes of Health in 1994 concluded that ". . . pharmacologic agents may be effective in reducing body weight over an extended period of time," and that, ". . . the drugs are effective and have a role in the treatment of obesity."

The *Harvard Heart Letter* cited a study in which phentermine and fenfluramine were combined with diet counseling and behavior modification. The patients averaged 200 pounds at the start of the study and lost, on average, over 30 pounds.

THE BIG LETDOWN

We fell in love with these drugs, and who can blame us? We even came up with a pet name for them: Phen-Fen. They were available, by prescription, through drugstores, weight-loss centers, the mail, and the Internet. Phen-Fen weight-loss programs were advertised on television, the radio, and in newspapers. I used the drugs extensively in my own medical weight-loss practice.

But the news wasn't all good. We knew from the beginning that Phen-Fen had side effects. Every medication does. A very small number of people in clinical trials, especially those taking higher doses, had complained of headaches, depression, sedation, excitation or insomnia, loose stools or constipation, blood-pressure elevation, dizziness, dry mouth, and a mild difficulty with concentration or memory that seemed to come and go.

By far the most serious, known potential side effect of these drugs, however, was PPH, or primary pulmonary hypertension. PPH is an elevation of blood pressure in the vessels that go from the heart to the lungs. It's a serious, often fatal condition that affects about one in a million people in the general population, usually a woman in her mid-thirties. The use of these two drugs raises that number.

Three to four people out of 100,000 who took these medications would contract the illness. About half of those would be reversible. In the remaining half, the patients would require heart–lung transplants to survive.

These were frightening statistics at first glance, but not nearly so frightening as the fact that over 300,000 people in the U.S. were dying each year from diseases associated with obesity. Other common drugs had worse side effects that occurred more frequently. The benefits, we felt, were worth the risk.

All that changed, however, when we saw the results of some small studies suggesting that fenfluramine and its close relative dexfenfluramine caused a side effect we had been completely unaware of: valvular heart disease. One group of researchers reported that as many as 30 percent of all people who used the drugs had developed some thickening of the valve that controls blood flow through the aorta, the heart's main blood vessel. This, obviously, could pose a grave danger to the health of these people.

The companies that manufactured the two drugs, commercially named Pondimin™ and Reduxt™, voluntarily recalled the products and immediately stopped producing them. Phentermine, commercially known as Ionamin™, never came into question. It is a very safe drug that is still in use today.

Since that initial research, no study has been able to duplicate the 30-percent figure, and many other studies have shown no significant rise in valvular disease with the use of these drugs. In my own practice, I saw neither PPH nor valvular disease in any of my patients—probably because I prescribed the drugs at only one quarter the recommended dosage (with great results). Still, we won't know for certain about safety until larger studies have been done. Until then, Phen-Fen will remain off the market.

THE PUZZLE WITHIN THE PUZZLE

Millions of overweight people across the country and in Europe felt unhappy and betrayed with Phen-Fen gone. The "Holy Grail" of weight loss—the key to the fat-storing switch—had been handed to them, then snatched away. The search was on to find a replacement. Phen-Fen showed us that throwing the switch was possible, but we had to find another way to do it.

Phen-Fen seemed to work for nearly everyone, so it was only natural to go looking for another drug, or combination of drugs, we could give to every patient who walked in the door. We tried Meridia® and orlistat, but neither showed the spectacular results we obtained with Phen-Fen.

Slowly, however, I began to notice something about my patients that started me thinking in a new direction. Although they all shared a similar problem—being overweight—their eating habits and the way they experienced hunger fell into four very distinct categories.

What was going on?

Here are profiles of four typical, but very different patients. See if you recognize yourself among them.

Anne Marie

Anne Marie is 38 years old, 5'5" tall, and weighs 180 pounds. She came to my office quite distraught telling me, "Dr. Rivas, I've tried everything to lose weight and just can't do it. I've read every diet book and tried every program. I'm always hungry and dieting. Also, when I eat I either don't get full or it takes a couple of hours for the fullness feeling to come. By then I'm absolutely stuffed and feel sick. Sometimes I don't get full at all, and an hour or two after a meal, I start eating all over again. In fact, I have to practically starve myself to lose anything at all. I even tried to exercise four times a week for the past month, but haven't lost one single pound. My family doctor told me that I am eating more than I admit and I just need to push myself away from the table and exercise more, but I swear, I'm always dieting! My metabolism must be dead. I have no energy so exercising is very hard, and sometimes I even feel slow mentally."

Mary Ann

Mary Ann presents a very different picture. She's a 42-year-old woman who has tried "absolutely everything but just can't lose weight." She has actually been exercising an hour a day and has been very careful about her fat consumption. Unfortunately, all her efforts have met with no success at all. She states quite emphatically that her

27

appetite is normal and that she doesn't think she feels unusually hungry most of the time. She does have very significant cravings for candy, cake, pies, and chocolates, however. "I know, even at the time, that I shouldn't eat them but I do anyway." She also admits to compulsive eating. This means that she eats even when she's not hungry, usually in response to stress, depression, loneliness, or boredom. On occasion, she may binge eat, or eat to great excess. She can be moody, often showing symptoms of PMS, and sometimes, especially during the winter, she becomes severely depressed.

Carla

Carla presents yet another picture. She's a 50 year old who's tried not only diets and exercise, but has used prescription medications, such as phentermine, and various natural weight-loss products as well. "I've lost about ten pounds and that's it," she says. She also feels listless and has no particular interest in doing anything. "I'm not sure if I'm depressed or just not enthused about anything. Nothing seems to excite me." She complains of craving fatty foods and chips, but sweets aren't really a problem.

Susan

Susan is 5'6" tall and weighs about 220 pounds. Her appetite is extremely well controlled and she isn't overeating, but her weight remains high. "This is so frustrating," she tells me. "For breakfast I'm eating a bagel with nothing on it; for lunch, a half a sandwich of fat-free turkey; and at dinner, I'm having fat-free pasta with a salad. For an evening snack I'll have a few pretzels. That's it for the entire day. It's impossible that I'm not losing any weight!"

WHAT'S GOING ON?

Here's what fascinated me: Each of the first three women's symptoms were typical of someone who was lacking a particular neurotransmitter. Anne Marie's constant hunger was a classic symptom of norepinephrine depletion. Mary Ann's bingeing indicated that her serotonin levels were obviously out of whack. Carla's listlessness and lack of interest in anything was a textbook picture of someone suffering from a dopamine deficiency.

Susan was another story. She was obviously *not* a case of neurotransmitter imbalance. What struck me about her daily fare was that it comprised mostly carbohydrates. I had run into this kind of patient before, even during the Phen-Fen days. Susan is a classic example of what I call the carbohydrate-sensitive individual. These people will not lose weight until their diets are free of starch and carbohydrates. I find this condition in about 5 percent of my patients. One man who came to me gained 55 pounds just by adding pretzels to his diet after having lost 70 pounds. Another has lost 65 pounds over 3 months by greatly limiting carbohydrate intake—he had lost only 5 pounds during the previous 3 months, despite eating very, very little.

BACK ON TRACK

If weight loss was a matter of targeting neurotransmitter imbalances, then throwing the switch would be easy! We already had safe and effective tools for doing that—and they weren't all prescription medications—some you could buy at the local health-food store. The best news of all, people would be able to lose weight with no effort whatsoever. Just throw the right switch, and the pounds would disappear on their own.

It was all simply a matter of figuring out which type of weight gainer you were.

I found that I could figure out each patient's type with about three minutes of conversation. Once I knew that, I could give them tools more powerful than Phen-Fen for getting down to a healthy, normal weight.

News from the Brain-Chemistry Front

Although we're very familiar with the effect serotonin, norepinephrine, and dopamine have on appetite, scientists are learning more about the brain chemistry of obesity every day. Within the past couple of years, researchers have discovered even more neurotransmitters (substances in the brain that cause cells to send an electrical message) that may affect the way you eat and gain weight.

Two of them, called hypocretin 1 and hypocretin 2, are located in the hypothalamus, a tiny part of the brain that controls food intake. They're similar in makeup to a hormone called secretin, which controls acid production in the stomach.

Although we're not sure yet exactly how these two substances control weight gain, their location in the brain tells us that they almost certainly have a profound effect.

IDENTIFYING YOUR TYPE

Here are the questions I ask each patient on his or her first visit. Answer them as accurately as you can, and you'll know your own type when you're finished.

Part 1

1. Do you have a large appetite?
   Do you almost always feel hungry?
   Can you eat almost anything
   in sight?. . . . . ☐ YES ☐ NO

2. Do you have a hard time
   getting full? Does it feel like
   you can just keep eating and
   eating? Is the feeling of fullness
   delayed, so that you've already
   eaten too much by the time
   the feeling of fullness occurs?
   Do you ever feel full at all?
   Do you even know what
   it means to be full?. . . . . ☐ YES ☐ NO

3. How is your energy level?
   Do you feel tired frequently
   and blame your exhaustion on
   your weight?. . . . . ☐ YES ☐ NO

4. Do you suspect that you have
   a slow metabolism? . . . . ☐ YES ☐ NO

5. Do you have trouble with
   motivation? . . . . ☐ YES ☐ NO

31

6. Do you have problems focusing
   on any one task? Are you scattered?
   Do you have symptoms of attention
   deficit disorder (ADD)? . . . . ☐ YES ☐ NO

7. Does your weight just seem to
   climb for no apparent reason
   or change of lifestyle? Are you
   out of control? Are both diet
   and exercise programs
   ineffective? . . . . ☐ YES ☐ NO

*If you answered "yes" to most of these questions, then
you have a norepinephrine-deficient brain-chemistry
type. Call yourself an* **N-Profile.**

Part 2

1. Are sweet cravings more of a
   problem than hunger? Is chocolate
   your weakness? Are cravings a
   significant problem at ovulation
   or menses? . . . . ☐ YES ☐ NO

2. Are you a compulsive eater?
   Do you eat in response to
   various stresses, that is,
   loneliness, boredom, anger,
   happiness, etc.? After you eat
   do you ask yourself why you
   just ate? . . . . ☐ YES ☐ NO

3. Do you binge? Do you find yourself
   eating very large quantities of food
   at one sitting? Do you eat so much
   at one time that you get nauseated? . . . ☐ YES ☐ NO

4. Are you obsessed by food? Is food on your mind through most of the day and may even awaken you at night? Are you up in the middle of the night eating? Are food thoughts driving you nuts? Is food too great a priority in your life? . . . . ☐ YES ☐ NO

5. Do you get depressed, moody, and irritable? Do you suffer with PMS? Do you have seasonal affective disorder or fibromyalgia? Do you suffer with migraines? . . . . . ☐ YES ☐ NO

6. Do you have a family history of alcoholism, depression, or PMS symptoms? . . . . ☐ YES ☐ NO

If you answered "yes" to most of these questions, then you are a serotonin-deficient brain-chemistry type. Call yourself an S-Profile.

Part 3

1. Do you continue to have cravings for salty or sweets even after various medications have been tried? . . . . . ☐ YES ☐ NO

2. Do you not enjoy life? Are you generally a "down" person? . . . . . . ☐ YES ☐ NO

3. Do you have an addictive personality? Do you need drugs to get high and forget your problems? . . . . ☐ YES ☐ NO

4. Are you easily distracted?. . . . . . . ☐ YES ☐ NO

5. Do you experience sexual
   dysfunction?. . . . . ☐ YES ☐ NO

*If you answer "yes" to most of these questions, then
you are a dopamine-deficient brain-chemistry type.
Call yourself a* **D-Profile***.*

Part 4

1. Are you unable to lose weight
   despite excellent appetite and
   craving control? . . . . ☐ YES ☐ NO

2. Are low-calorie diets ineffective? . . . ☐ YES ☐ NO

3. Does exercise cause no weight
   loss at all? . . . . ☐ YES ☐ NO

4. Do medications fail to help you?. . . . ☐ YES ☐ NO

5. Do you tend to eat mainly
   carbohydrates such as breads,
   pasta, fruits, etc.? . . . . ☐ YES ☐ NO

*If you answer "yes" to most of these questions,
then you are carbohydrate sensitive. Call yourself a*
C-Profile*.*

That's all there is to it! Now you have all the basic
understanding you'll need to throw the switch and start losing weight.

4

N-Profile:
The Universal Type

If you have an N-Profile, you're in good company. Norepi-nephrine deficiency is by far the most common weight-loss challenge I see in my practice. But N-Profiles aren't the only people who suffer with the problem. *Everyone* who is overweight, to some extent, needs to raise his or her norepinephrine level. That's why *it's important that you read this chapter no matter what your profile.*

If you're lucky enough to be an N-Profile—the simplest and easiest to treat—raising your norepinephrine level is the only step you'll need to take to lose weight. If you have a different profile, however, you should also read all chapters that specifically apply to you.

Joanne's Story

When Joanne first came to my office, she was 27 years old, 5'4" tall, 190 pounds, and beginning to feel as if her difficulty in losing weight would drive her over the edge of sanity.

When she sat down across from me in my consultation room, she looked distraught and tired.

At one time or other, she told me, she had tried practically every fad diet program on the market, from those that offer weekly weigh-in meetings to those that restrict you to mail-order food—which they're happy to provide at a premium price. None of them worked. Her hunger was too strong.

"I can't stop eating," she said. "I'm always hungry and my appetite is unbelievable. I don't even know what being full feels like."

To make matters worse, she wasn't burning up many of those extra calories through physical activity. She felt too tired to exercise. Sometimes, in desperation, she forced herself to ignore her insatiable appetite and restrict her food intake to levels that would frighten a fasting monk. Unfortunately, that didn't work any better than the fad diets had.

She felt she had come to the end of the road, where her weight was concerned, but in fact, she hadn't. She had simply, finally, made the right turn.

THE N-PROFILE'S PROFILE

Literally thousands of people have come to my office reciting almost exactly the same tale of frustration and disappointment. Often a patient will confide that she has other family members who suffer from similar weight problems—or just as telling, from attention disorders. She may have been quite thin for most of her life, then watched in horror as her dress size suddenly began to increase in an uncontrollable way. Her energy level has slipped into the doldrums, a fact she attributes to her weight and poor metabolism. She is clearly depressed, and she even complains about having difficulty concentrating and focusing.

Here are the main symptoms to look for. If you have two or more of them, then the norepinephrine level in your brain is probably out of balance.

Hunger

As with Joanne, the most prominent symptom of the typical N-Profile person is increased appetite. Often you'll feel hungry through most of the day, but you'll feel absolutely famished in the late afternoons and evenings. Typical N-Profile hunger demands "real foods" rather than junk foods.

Insatiability

As an N-Profile person, you do not always overeat, but always want to. You may complain that you "never feel full" during meals and don't know when to stop eating, so you'll just choose some arbitrary moment to quit the table. You may never feel full, or the feeling may hit you two to three hours later, when you'll find yourself feeling absolutely stuffed. The feeling that you're full is called *satiety*. So if you can't achieve that feeling, you're literally insatiable.

Cravings

You may also have cravings but most often for starches, like breads and pastas, rather than sweets, and the feelings are occasional rather than constant. Some people mistake cravings for hunger, but there is a difference. A craving is a very strong desire for a particular food that cannot be satisfied by anything else. Hunger is more general and nonspecific.

Those Norepinephrine Blues

Many people complain that they wake up tired and can't get themselves moving all day. They often suspect, erroneously, that their thyroid is out of whack. Other people seem "okay" in the morning, but generally burn out with fatigue as the day goes on. These are the folks you'll see taking afternoon naps.

All of this fatigue can come with some jitteriness and shakiness, which is often blamed—again erroneously—on a drop in their blood sugar or a hypoglycemic event.

Amazingly, these symptoms almost always completely resolve after raising the brain's norepinephrine levels. The patients feel great throughout the whole day and evening. All of this suggests that their symptoms were actually from low norepinephrine levels, not from low sugar levels or hypothyroidism at all.

Exhaustion

You may have low energy levels, but this has nothing to do with low metabolism. It's because your brain's norepinephrine level is low. Norepinephrine is very similar to adrenaline, often called the "fight or flight" transmitter. Both substances are potent mental and physical energizers, so it's not at all surprising that a person with an N-Profile will often feel "blah."

Attention Difficulties

As an N-Profile, you often, but not always, complain you have poor focus and concentration. One of my patients is a business executive and owner of a very large company. He told me how difficult it used to be for him to run his business effectively because his mind was always wandering. Because his ability to concentrate on a single issue was poor, at times so was his memory. After his norepinephrine levels were restored to balance, he was like a different person. Now his business is booming and, as an added bonus, his interaction with his family has improved. He is a much more patient listener and much more efficient at everything he does. If this sounds like attention deficit disorder (ADD), it's because it is. What we commonly refer to as ADD is most certainly nothing more than a neurotransmitter deficiency, which can be easily corrected in most instances. When there is a coexisting weight problem, it is easy to correct both at once.

Depression

You may experience some depression—not usually profound, but bad enough to interfere with daily life. Often you won't realize how "down" you really are until you've thrown your norepinephrine switch and notice at once how light your spirit has become.

MEDICAL TREATMENT

Because the N-Profile is the most common type, it's also the easiest to treat. Simply raising norepinephrine levels will reset the brain thermostat and turn off the hunger switch, so that weight loss begins to happen automatically and effort-

> ### The N-Profile at a Glance
>
> *Symptoms:*
>
> ☐ Hunger
> ☐ Insatiability
> ☐ Cravings for starchy foods
> ☐ Depression
> ☐ Exhaustion
> ☐ Attention deficit

lessly. You can do this with either over-the-counter supplements or with prescription medication; but phentermine, a medication, is easily the best tool we have. Virtually everyone in the field agrees. (But in either case—whether you take the prescription medication or supplements— you should consult a physician before embarking on a weight-loss regimen.)

Again, although phentermine is part of the Phen-Fen combination, it has absolutely nothing to do with causing heart valve problems or pulmonary hypertension. All those health concerns are side effects of fenfluramine, *not* phentermine. Phentermine has been on the market for over 40 years and has proven extremely safe. In my practice, over 10,000 people have used the drug without experiencing any significant long-term side effects. In fact, I'll go out on a limb and say that it's probably the safest thing I use for any condition.

People usually feel the effect of the medication with the first dose. They marvel at how their weight starts to drop and hunger disappears, and how they generally feel more energized and focused. "Miracle" is the word I hear most often to describe this effect.

The usual weight loss is 5–10 pounds over the first two weeks. People who lose less than 4 pounds over this period need to either increase their dose or add another medication to their regimen. After an initial fast start, weight loss should settle down to about 1–2 pounds per week.

Remember, the rate at which you lose fat is very much determined by your brain thermostat—*not* by diet, exercise, or metabolism. For the most part, you'll find yourself a spectator watching the number on the scale go down week by week, until it just stops.

When you finally stop losing you will have reached your new set point. You'll know you're there because your weight will remain the same for 3–6 weeks no matter what changes you make in your medication. It's almost impossible to lose any more weight past this new set point. If you follow the program, you'll probably remain within a few pounds of this weight for the rest of your life.

Side Effects

The most common side effects I see are dry mouth, insomnia for the first night or two, and occasionally nervousness for the first day. Constipation is sometimes a complaint, but you can relieve it easily by using a fiber supplement and drinking more fluids. On very rare occasions, a patient may experience some tongue soreness or headaches.

All of these side effects are usually mild and tolerable, and hardly ever cause people to go off their program. (But if you have any side effects at all, be sure to tell your doctor.)

Phentermine is safe to use with most other medications, but before you begin this regimen, make a list of any other medications you're taking, and tell your physician. I advise patients not to use phentermine with decongestants like Sudafed® or phenylpropanolamine. Also, *never* use it with MAO inhibitors such as Nardil®.

How to Use Phentermine

When first taking phentermine, most people start on a 37.5-mg tablet at 11 a.m. every day. You should take it on an empty stomach, so eat breakfast before 9 a.m. and lunch after 12 noon. I prefer tablets because they can be broken and are easier to tolerate. Some people do better with half a pill at 11 a.m. and another half at 4 p.m., since evening hunger is often the major problem. I have safely taken scores of patients up to two tablets a day without any significant problems.

As for problems with addiction, there is no evidence that it will cause dependency, even among people who have used it for many years. There are no cravings for the drug and no withdrawal. There is certainly no sense of euphoria.

Follow your physician's instructions when you're taking phentermine. This medication should not be used by pregnant or lactating women, or by people with untreated glaucoma, heart disease, or uncontrolled hypertension. However, I have had many patients with controlled hypertension whose blood pressure normalized with weight loss.

Men with untreated enlargement of the prostate should also be careful about its use, as it may make the problem worse. If you have this problem and you're using phentermine, be sure to stay in close contact with your doctor.

In the Long Term

Some patients are able to take phentermine for years without developing any tolerance—which means that their bodies don't grow used to the drug and make it ineffective. For others, however, the medication loses some of its effectiveness and hunger begins to return after about six months.

This is a signal that the brain chemistry is becoming unbalanced once again, and the thermostat, now moving up, has thrown the hunger switch back on. At this point, you'll need to consult with your doctor about adding another norepinephrine-releasing agent to regain the proper chemical balance.

The best choice is usually phendimetrazine at 35 mg twice a day or a 75-mg dose pack of another drug called Tenuate® at 4 P.M. These are added to the prior dose of phentermine.

Another good approach is to add a 500-mg dose of the amino acid tyrosine (available at your local health-food store) to the phentermine.

The side effects of these other agents are similar to those of phentermine.

Obviously, a physician must prescribe these medications, and he or she must be quite familiar with their use. A specialist in bariatrics (weight control) is preferable.

Some patients, however, prefer an all-natural approach to prescription medications. There's plenty of hope for them as well.

NATURAL TREATMENT

While medicines remain the best way to increase brain neurotransmitters and turn off the hunger switch, some people are reluctant to use them. In fact, quite a few of the people who come to me for treatment hesitate to take even an aspirin for a headache. Just waving a prescription pad in their direction would send them fleeing from my office.

Fortunately, I can keep my pad in my pocket. There are some natural supplements that can be extremely effective at turning off the hunger switch, so long as they're used properly—which means taking them in the proper dosage, at the right times of day, and in the proper combination.

A Powerful Combination

The most effective—and most controversial—natural treatment for weight loss is the combination of ephedra with caffeine. Most often this appears on the label as Ma Huang with Guarana.

Okay, before you shake your head, wag your finger, and say, "But all the reporters on the six o'clock news are warning us NOT to use ephedra," consider this: Ma Huang has been used safely by the Chinese for thousands of years as an energizer and weight-loss enhancer. Actually, it's also been sitting on store shelves in the U.S. for a long time, but only recently has it become controversial. Why? Mostly because a product called Metabolife®, which includes ephedra as one of its active ingredients, has put it into the public spotlight.

Over the past several years, millions of bottles of Metabolife® and other, similar products have been sold in the U.S. and other parts of the world. Of course, the inevitable happened. Reports of problems began to surface, as they do whenever large numbers of unsupervised people start ingesting any substance that's stronger than a sugar pill. Even commonplace foods such as shellfish, peanuts, and chocolate often cause allergic reactions, which are sometimes so powerful they can become life threatening. So it would come as no surprise if ephedra turned out to be a danger to the public health. But is it?

44

For three years now, the FDA has unsuccessfully attempted to limit the use of ephedra products due to adverse event reports, and for three years, it has been unsuccessful. The reason: No one has been able to prove a causal relationship between the adverse effects and ephedra. (For details about the legal aspects of this controversy, be sure to read the Afterword by attorney James R. Prochnow, J.D., beginning on page 145.)

What's going on? Are people simply imagining things? Upon close inspection, it appears that most of the reported problems arose when consumers deliberately overdosed themselves, ignored warnings about drug interactions and preexisting medical conditions, or in some other way misused the substance. To complicate matters even further, the FDA has used very poor techniques in gathering its data—which is why Congress has rejected the FDA's request to limit sale of the substance.

In one case, for example, the FDA reported that an 18-year-old male committed suicide while using ephedra. It would be easy to make the assumption that ephedra caused him to suffer a depression, which led to his death. However, an autopsy revealed that the young man had both ephedrine and *codeine*, a controlled narcotic, in his blood. There was no data whatsoever offered on the source, dose, or length and frequency of the man's use of ephedra.

In another case, a 30-year-old female died in the middle of the night in a car accident. She had been speeding at 90 mph in the wrong direction on a one-way street. She ran a stop sign and hit a tree. An autopsy showed ephedrine and caffeine in her blood, so, of course, they had to be the culprits behind her risky behavior. Except that the same autopsy showed the presence of pseudo-ephedrine (an over-the-counter antihistamine) in her blood, as well as an alcohol level of .212 %!

In other cases, one woman claimed ephedra caused her Norplant contraceptive device to fail, and was thus responsible for her pregnancy. Another blamed ephedra for excess nose and body hair.

To put all this in better perspective, in 1999 there were 25 reported significant adverse reactions out of 3 *billion* servings of ephedra. This is an incredibly low incidence. By those statistics certainly almost any ingested substance is more dangerous. My patients have used ephedra/caffeine (EC) with great success and no serious problems.

As Effective as Prescription Medication

There is no question that ephedra/caffeine is effective at turning off the hunger switch. A very well-designed, controlled study in Denmark of subjects using EC over a 6-month period showed an average weight loss of 37.4 pounds. Another study concluded that EC is more effective than the old weight-control drug Redux®.

EC is also unique in that it encourages the body to burn fat rather than muscle, unlike most diets, which cause significant muscle wasting. Furthermore, EC seems to target belly fat, which is the most dangerous form. Also, unlike some medications, EC does not seem to lose its potency over time. It remains very effective after months of daily use.

EC also has two significant advantages over and above weight loss. It increases concentration and energy, and it raises HDL cholesterol levels (the good kind that protects your arteries).

Its mechanism of action is rather clear. Ephedrine increases release of norepinephrine in the brain similar to phentermine. Caffeine inhibits the breakdown of norepi-nephrine. So norepinephrine levels go up, the brain chem-istry has a better balance, the thermostat goes down, the switch goes off, and weight loss ensues.

How to Use EC

Dosage is very important both for effectiveness and safety.

The total dose of ephedra should probably not exceed 48 mg per day, though there aren't many studies to support this statement. This is my experienced opinion. I also prefer tablets, as they can be broken in half.

Ephedra usually comes in the form of the Chinese herb Ma Huang, but it may also simply be labeled as ephedra. I prefer my patients to use yet another form, called country mallow, although it's much harder to find.

Start with one half of a 12-mg tablet at 11 A.M. and 4 P.M. If you tolerate this dose well and you haven't noticed any change in your feelings of hunger, you can go up to one tablet twice a day. If you need to, you can go higher, but max out at two tablets twice a day.

Side effects, which are similar to those of caffeine, often appear after the initial dose, but diminish after continued use. They include mild nervousness, insomnia, agitation, and a slight rise in blood pressure. People with heart disease, untreated hypertension, anxiety disorders, or prostate enlarge-ment should avoid ephedra. As always, you should keep your doctor informed of the supplements and medications you're taking, and let your physician know about side effects.

Medications that should not be taken with ephedra products include MAO inhibitors (i.e., Nardil®, clonidine, and yohimbine). If you're taking decongestants, stop using ephedra immediately if you notice any unusual side effects.

It's important to note that ephedra alone is not very effective in causing weight loss. You need to combine it with a caffeine product such as guarana or my current favorite, green tea extract.

Green tea contains two main active ingredients, catechins and caffeine, both of which lead to norepinephrine release. The catechins in green tea help to rein in an enzyme called COMT, which breaks down norepinephrine. The caffeine does the same thing to an enzyme called phosphodiesterase, which again leads to higher norepinephrine levels.

Recent studies set the effective dose at 50 mg of caffeine and 90 mg of catechin taken three times a day with meals. The catechins work best in the form of *epigallo catechin gallate;* unfortunately, containers don't always carry this information. I recommend taking 200 mg of green tea extract twice a day.

Green tea has another benefit, by the way: It may reduce the risk of a heart attack by 45 percent.

Tyrosine Can Help

A much lesser known, but very effective natural product is the amino acid L-tyrosine, or tyrosine for short. Combining it with ephedra can reduce appetite by 50 percent more than by using ephedra alone.

This intriguing amino acid raises both dopamine and norepinephrine levels. It has been found useful in treating attention deficit problems, addictions, fatigue, narcolepsy, depression, and sexual dysfunction.

Its effects on reducing stress are rather striking. Studies done by the U.S. military show a significant reduction in combat fatigue and battle stress among those taking L-tyrosine supplements. In yet another study, tyrosine increased cognitive performance, improved mood, and sped up reaction time of the subjects.

Its effect on appetite and in regulating brain chemistry works best when it's combined with other agents, such as phentermine. Doses of 500 mg to 2,000 mg per day are quite safe and effective. For my patients who prefer natural substances to pharmaceuticals, I have combined country mallow with green tea extract and tyrosine with very good results. Let your doctor know if you're taking tyrosine. As with almost everything else, it shouldn't be taken with MAO inhibitors.

Where to Find L-tyrosine

L-tyrosine is a naturally occurring food component that balances brain chemistry by raising norepinephrine and dopamine levels. It seems beneficial for improving mental performance, reducing stress, overcoming addictions, elevating mood, and increasing sex drive. In conjunction with other agents, it can also turn back the thermostat in the brain, flip the hunger switch, and reduce weight.

One way to help increase the l-tyrosine levels in your brain is by getting more from the foods you eat. Here are the top picks for tyrosine-rich foods:

Wheat germ	Chicken
Ricotta	Turkey
Cottage cheese	Duck
Pork	Wild game

5

S-Profile: The Depression Connection

Serotonin is another, very powerful neurotransmitter, which your brain uses to control mood, emotions, aggressiveness, sleep, and appetite. A low level can do more than cause you to gain weight; it can also plunge you into the deepest, blackest depression.

We've known about the connection between being overweight and depression for a long time. In fact, the first side effect researchers noticed when they began studying fluoxin (Prozac®) was that it sometimes caused weight loss. This drug, of course, is aimed directly at raising serotonin levels in the brain.

THE S-PROFILE'S PROFILE

S-Profiles, people who are serotonin deficient, are the second most common type of weight gainer. Very often they share some characteristics with N-Profiles, but their serotonin symptoms are far more powerful. Here's what to look for.

Cravings

If you have an S-Profile, then you know the meaning of the word "craving," especially where sweets are concerned. Pastries, cookies, and candy seem to reach out and touch you. Chocolate—oh, that wonderful chocolate—holds more allure than gold. Otherwise, you may have a perfectly normal appetite. You don't feel hunger is your constant companion, and meals make you feel full, as they should. You probably have no problem with any food type other than sweets.

Cravings are not a minor problem. In fact, they can be completely overwhelming. One of my patients described how she used to awaken in the mornings surrounded by empty candy bar wrappers. She had no idea she had even eaten the candy during the night.

Compulsive Eating

Another common symptom of the S-Profile patient is eating without hunger, most often in response to stress or uncomfortable emotions. You may find yourself eating when you're depressed, bored, anxious, or lonely. You may not even realize that you're eating. An S-Profile person often munches unconsciously. Then after you've finished, you suddenly become aware that you've consumed the equivalent of an entire meal—a meal you really didn't want.

Food Obsession

Sometimes you just can't get food off your mind. In fact, food is all you think about. This then leads to irrational, ritualistic eating behaviors, over which you seem to have little or no control. This is similar to an obsession with cleanliness that leads to compulsive hand washing. People will wash their hands to the point of scrubbing off layers of skin, even though they know that what they are doing makes no sense and that it is hurting them. They just cannot help themselves.

Binge Eating

This is an extremely exaggerated form of compulsive eating and/or craving. You may eat an enormous quantity at one sitting and feel quite ill afterward. Episodes may be either common or rare, but they tend to come and go.

Depression

It's not unusual for an S-Profile person to have a history of depression or to have used antidepressant medication. Often, you will complain that your depression is linked to your weight, but actually it's a separate issue. The good news, however, is that you can clear up both problems at the same time.

Anxiety and Panic Attacks

Anxiety is a feeling of vague uneasiness or apprehension over nothing in particular. It can be either mild and tolerable or quite severe. Sometimes it can generate panic attacks. Severe and often disabling, these attacks can overwhelm you

> **The S-Profile at a Glance**
>
> *Symptoms:*
>
> ❑ Cravings
> ❑ Compulsive eating
> ❑ Food obsession
> ❑ Binge eating
> ❑ Depression
> ❑ Anxiety and panic attacks
> ❑ Phobias

with feelings of pain, shortness of breath, sweating, shakiness, and nervousness.

Phobias

If you've ever had an irrational fear of anything at all that stops you in your tracks and seems to completely immobilize you, then you know the meaning of the word "phobia." Whether you're afraid of heights, crowds, small spaces, or spiders, the panic and paralysis is the same, and it's due largely to a deficiency of serotonin.

MEDICAL TREATMENT

Treating the symptoms of an S-Profile involves raising the brain's serotonin levels, but if you're trying to lose weight, it's not a good idea to take a serotonin drug by itself. When taken alone, serotonin medications almost always make you *gain* weight, rather than lose it. This is particularly true, I have found, for the antidepressant Paxil®. On the other hand, these agents can be extremely effective when combined with the norepinephrine-releasing agents, which were discussed in the previous chapter. *(If you haven't read the N-Profile chapter, take the time to do so now. Nearly everyone with a weight problem suffers from some degree of norepinephrine deficiency.)*

Serotonin medications must be prescribed by a doctor, and you'll want to keep your physician well-informed about the effects of these drugs. My favorite combination for S-Profile people is phentermine with Effexor® XR. The XR form of Effexor® is a slow-release capsule, which is good for 24 hours and has very few associated side effects. It is crucial to keep the dose low: *a 37.5-mg dose once a day with food.* This, combined with 30 mg of phentermine can be extremely effective at stopping sweet cravings, binges, and compulsive eating. It will also greatly help with anxiety, depression, and

Serotonin Drugs Made Easy

It's important to understand how serotonin drugs work. They are, as a group, called selective serotonin reuptake inhibitors (SSRIs). These agents don't add serotonin to the brain. Instead, they prevent the "breakdown" and reabsorbtion of serotonin that's already there, creating a sort of reservoir that slowly fills up. It's similar to putting a plug into the drain of a sink and allowing the water from a dripping faucet to gradually accumulate in the bowl. Because they don't cause the brain to manufacture extra serotonin, the SSRIs, as a class, have proven over a long period of time to be extremely safe as well as effective.

Maybe the most well-known medication of this type is Prozac®, which revolutionized the treatment of depression. Other drugs, used for the same purpose, include Zoloft®, Paxil®, Effexor®, and Serzone®. Another SSRI, Meridia®, works in the same way, but targets cells that specifically affect hunger.

moodiness. I prefer Effexor® over other SSRIs because it causes an accumulation in the brain of both serotonin and norepinephrine, thereby helping to balance both chemistries and lead to an even greater response.

The side effects I see most frequently are headache and occasional fatigue. Very rarely, patients experience sexual dysfunction. As always, if you have any side effects, you should tell your doctor.

It is always important to keep the doses as low as possible since more is definitely not better.

The other combination, which can be very useful, is phentermine with 10 mg of Prozac®. This is especially good for patients who may get a headache from Effexor®. Dr. Michael Anchors discusses this therapy in great detail in his book *Safer Than Phen-Fen.*

If these combinations begin to lose their effectiveness, you can consult your doctor about using a combination of 10 mg of the amino acid 5-hydroxytryptophan with 5 mg of carbidopa. This is a prescription compound that only a pharmacist can make. Take the first dose before bed, then twice a day thereafter if you need to. Dr. Richard Rothman of the National Institutes of Health uses this combination widely and with good success. Remember, it is to be added to, *not* substituted for, your other medications.

Another, relatively new drug that treats serotonin deficiency is Meridia®. It, too, acts as an SSRI and increases both norepinephrine and serotonin levels in the brain. When used by itself, it seems only mildly effective, but it works extremely well when combined with phentermine for the S-Profile patient. It has also proven remarkably safe among the patients who have used it in my practice. The package carries a warning that a small percentage of people may experience a rise in blood pressure, but none of my patients have experienced this problem. If you do experience any side effects, however, tell your doctor right away.

NATURAL TREATMENT

Several natural products will elevate serotonin levels. To maximize their effect, however, you'll need to use them with norepinephrine-raising supplements.

The best supplement for raising serotonin levels is tryptophan, an amino acid, which consumers once used extensively as a sleep-inducing agent. Unfortunately, a fatal outbreak in 1989 of a rare autoimmune disease called eosinophilia myalgia syndrome (EMS) was associated with the use of tryptophan. The gathered evidence clearly pointed to a contaminant in the processing plant of one Japanese manufacturer. Since then the FDA has banned its use as an over-the-counter supplement.

Prior to this contamination, people all over the world used tryptophan for many years without incident. Since there doesn't seem to be a problem with tryptophan itself, it's unclear why it wasn't allowed back on store shelves once the contamination issue was resolved. As of 1996, you can once again buy tryptophan, but you need a doctor's prescription. Bring the prescription to a compounding pharmacist (one who mixes compounds).

Effective doses range from 500 mg to 2,000 mg a day. For the best effect, you can take tryptophan at night and tyrosine in the morning.

If you don't want to go to the trouble of getting a prescription filled, you can purchase a product called 5-HTP (5-hydroxytryptophan) over the counter. It also raises serotonin levels. Many doctors have used it successfully, and some stud-

Tasty Tryptophan

The FDA may have taken tryptophan off of drugstore shelves, but you can still find it at your local supermarket. Plenty of delicious foods can add tryptophan to your diet. Generally turkey and milk are good sources. Here is a list of other foods that contain tryptophan:

Wheat germ	Avocado
Cottage cheese	Ham
Pork	Eggs
Luncheon meat	Almonds
Duck	

ies have proven its effectiveness in treating depression as well as obesity. I know of physicians who also use it for fibromyalgia and allergies. It's even used to help control anger, irritability, and anxiety.

One study looked at overweight diabetics who took 5-HTP in very large doses (250 mg three times a day). The subjects who used the supplement lost an average of 4.6 pounds more than did the subjects who were given sugar pills. Another study showed a 5-percent weight loss over 12 weeks among subjects who took a dose of 200–300 mg before meals.

The results of both studies were affected by a common side effect of the supplement: nausea. I have also seen a fair amount of nausea associated with this supplement, especially when it's taken with Effexor®, so I would avoid that particular combination. Nausea tends to go away by the second week of using 5-HTP.

I prefer a sublingual spray of 10 mg per spray, which bypasses the GI tract and thereby avoids any nausea. The spray works in about two minutes, as compared with 15 minutes for a capsule. The spray can be used on an as-needed basis and is especially effective in curbing sweet cravings.

As with any substance that raises serotonin, to make a significant impact on weight loss, you should use 5-HTP in combination with N-Profile agents, such as ephedra–caffeine products or phentermine. Take them as you normally would, and use the 5-HTP spray as needed throughout the day. Dr. Michael Murray, the author of a book on 5-HTP, gets an average weight loss of a pound a week using 50–100 grams in supplement form three times a day, 20 minutes before meals. He also finds it useful for depression and fibromyalgia. If nausea becomes a problem, ginger tea may help.

6

D-Profile: The Root of All Pleasure

Researchers have a theory. They believe—at least many of them do—that every pleasurable feeling we have, from excitement of sex to the ecstasy of listening to a symphonic masterpiece, funnels through the dopamine system in the brain. Dopamine, like norepinephrine and serotonin, is a potent neurotransmitter, and the message it transmits from cell to cell is pleasure. One of its other jobs is closely related. It not only allows you to feel pleasure, but it drives you to seek it out.

The more dopamine you make, the better you feel. Of course, the opposite is also true. The less you make, the more blah your day is likely to be. If you're too low on the stuff, that last symphony or romantic encounter felt . . . well . . . okay, but not really wonderful. In fact, if you're low on dopamine, everything feels sort of okay, but never any better than that.

If that sounds like a description of your own experience, then you may have a D-Profile.

PORTRAIT OF A D-PROFILE

Sometimes the best clue for recognizing if you're a person with a D-Profile is that you don't respond to treatments for norepinephrine and serotonin depletion. In other words, it's a process of elimination. Or perhaps you started to lose weight on those other treatments, but then suddenly stopped—until a treatment that raised your level of dopamine kick-started your fat-burning engine into overdrive.

If you take a close look at yourself, you should be able to recognize your own D-Profile by the common characteristics listed below.

Depression

The neurotransmitter dopamine is responsible for the "natural highs" that people experience. The high of winning sports competition, or getting a good grade in school, or a promotion at work all originate with dopamine.

Therefore, if you have a depletion of this transmitter, you may feel generally down, or depressed, or just blah. You have a hard time getting motivated or enjoying the pleasures of everyday life. This could lead to the extreme of a rather severe depression.

Addictive Personality

Alcohol, tobacco, and many dangerous "street drugs" can stimulate dopamine release, which is what makes them so addictive. People who are especially sensitive to these substances probably have an unusually strong "dopaminergic" response because their basic levels are low. This is most likely the foundation in the brain for the so-called "addictive personality." This is often the hallmark of a person with a D-Profile. If you find that you can easily make a habit of taking substances that give you pleasure, or if you have a strong family history of addictions, then you may find that raising your dopamine levels will help you lose weight.

The Obesity–Cocaine Connection

Cocaine, carbohydrates, and fatty foods may all have something in common: They may all increase the level of dopamine in the brain, thereby leading to addiction in the case of the drug, or obesity in the case of the foods.

Cocaine is the most powerful dopamine-raising agent we know of. By dramatically increasing the level of dopamine available to synapses in the pleasure center of the brain, called the *nucleus accumbens*, it rewards the user with tremendous rushes of pleasure that "teach" the cells to hunger after more cocaine. Carbohydrates, while not nearly so powerful, can have a similar effect. When we consume lots of rice or pasta in response to a craving, we may simply be reacting to signals, sent by brain cells, requesting higher levels of dopamine. Wellbutrin®, SAMe, phenylalinine, and l-tyrosine all give higher levels, but keep them within a safety zone—and they don't bring a lot of fat or calories with them.

> ## The D-Profile at a Glance
>
> *Symptoms:*
>
> ☐ Depression
>
> ☐ Addictive personality
>
> ☐ Sexual dysfunction
>
> ☐ Specialized cravings

Sexual Dysfunction

Since dopamine is what allows you to experience the pleasure of orgasm, a low level may lead to sexual problems. You might experience delayed orgasm or even the inability to have an orgasm at all. Or you may simply find that your sexual desire has dwindled like a candle flame running out of wick.

Unfortunately, people often live with this kind of problem for years without recognizing its cause. They may blame themselves or their partners. Or sometimes their partners may be very angry with them for their lack of sexual interest or response.

Specialized Cravings

Strong desire for either fatty or salty foods is another D-Profile signpost. You tend to love bacon, sausage, steak, and other high-fat treats. A craving for starches is also common. So you may show a strong desire for potato chips, corn chips, or salted and buttered popcorn.

MEDICAL TREATMENT

Absolutely the best drug for anyone with a D-Profile is the prescription drug Wellbutrin®. Wellbutrin® is also used to

The Satiety Substance

Researchers at the Yerkes Primate Research Center of Emory University in Atlanta published in 1998 the results of a study that revealed yet another connection between cocaine and appetite. While looking at the effects of cocaine on the brain, scientists discovered a new neurotransmitter that seemed to regulate the feeling of fullness you get when you've eaten enough. They called the substance Cocaine and Amphetamine Transcript (CART) because it seemed to increase in the brains of rodents that had been given cocaine. The researchers discovered that when the substance was present in high levels the rodents lost their appetite. When amounts were low, their appetite increased. These results helped explain why cocaine and amphetamines had such a dramatic weight-loss affect on users. In the future, these studies may help scientists to develop safer and more effective drugs in the treatment of obesity.

treat depression and to help people quit smoking, so it obviously has a strong effect on the dopamine system.

As for how much to take and how often, your doctor may prescribe 150 mg of Wellbutrin® SR once every 12 hours. This seems to be a low, safe, effective dose.

Wellbutrin® acts in much the same way an SSRI drug does. It causes an accumulation of dopamine in the brain by preventing its rapid reabsorbtion, but it does not make your brain manufacture more of the stuff. That's why it's non-addicting.

Once again, your doctor should have you take Wellbutrin® with N-Profile and/or S-Profile agents to be effective. (If you haven't read the N-Profile chapter, you should take a look at it now.) It is not particularly useful by itself.

Phentermine and Wellbutrin® work well together, and adding Effexor® as a third ingredient works even more effectively. I have found this combination to be extremely well-tolerated, with few, if any, side effects. Occasionally, someone will feel overexcited after the initial dose, but the effect usually subsides quickly with continued use. If you notice any side effects, infrom your doctor.

After starting treatment with Wellbutrin®, patients with a D-Profile often report to me that their cravings are gone in a couple of days or even sooner. It's also common to feel a surge of energy and well-being shortly after beginning therapy.

Unfortunately, if you have a history of epilepsy or seizures, you won't be able to use this drug. There are, however, safe and effective natural supplements that can do almost as good a job. Be sure your doctor knows your full medical history before you begin this medication.

NATURAL TREATMENT

If you've kept up at all with the news in the world of natural medicine, you've heard about a particular amino acid called SAMe (s-adenosyl L-methionine). It has become a popular remedy for treating arthritis and depression.

Researchers have found that L-methionine raises dopamine, norepinephrine, and serotonin. It comes as a supplement and is also found in certain foods such as sunflower seeds.

If you take SAMe, tell your doctor. It's important to use vitamin B_6 along with it to prevent SAMe from converting into homocysteine, a substance that can increase your risk of heart disease. As an antidepressant, methionine has proven as effective as many prescription medications in clinical trials. It appears to be very safe, even at large doses, especially when taken with vitamin B_6. You can take 1 to 3 grams of methionine per day.

Another amino acid, phenylalanine, which is a "precursor" of tyrosine in the body, elevates both dopamine and norepinephrine and helps to keep them in balance.

In addition to weight loss, phenylalanine has been used effectively for depression at 200 mg a day and is better absorbed than tyrosine. It can be a rather effective pain reliever and can be used for PMS symptoms. It's highly concentrated in meats and cottage cheese. You can take up to 8 grams per day in supplement form.

People can't take phenylalanine if they have PKU (phenylketonuria), which is a rare illness affecting 1 in 40,000 people.

7

C-Profile: When Pasta Is the Problem

Medical science is full of mysteries. We don't really understand how some people spontaneously recover from incurable diseases, why some people become mentally ill, or what triggers a person to start putting on weight by so much as tasting a slice of white bread. Yet these things happen.

Yes, there are people whose brain chemistry is so sensitive to the effects of carbohydrates that they absolutely will not lose any significant amount of weight unless they severely reduce their carbohydrate intake. This is the essence of the C-Profile.

What are carbohydrates? To put it simply, starches and sugars. Rice, beans, bread, pretzels, corn, potatoes, white sugar, brown sugar, honey, pasta—some of our very favorite foods—all fall into the category.

THE C-PROFILE'S PROFILE

The C-Profile weight gainer is typically the most difficult to diagnose. About 1 in 5 of my patients shows an oversensitivity to carbohydrates, so it's not a terribly unusual condition. What makes it so difficult to diagnose is that it displays no easy-to-spot symptoms. Generally, I'll make the diagnosis simply by excluding all other possibilities.

Here's what generally happens. On her initial visit, a patient—we'll call her Julie—will seem to present the symptoms of a mixed type. Maybe she has a strong appetite, some cravings for carbohydrates, and her mood seems generally blah. I'll first give her a combination of medications to turn off cravings, decrease appetite, and increase fullness.

At this point, the typical person would easily lose weight because his or her brain chemistry is in balance and the thermostat is pushed back. But in Julie's case, the weight seems to cling to her stubbornly, despite an absence of cravings, compulsive eating, or ravenous appetite. No combination of medications or supplements leads to weight loss. There is only one conclusion left: She has a type of extreme carbohydrate sensitivity that makes it extremely easy for her to gain weight and difficult for her to lose it.

The C-Profile at a Glance

Symptoms:

☐ Mixed symptoms from the other profiles

☐ Failure to respond to drugs or natural supplements

☐ Quick weight response to lowering or raising of dietary carbohydrates

CARB ADDICTION?

You don't have to be a "carbohydrate addict" to have a C-Profile. Maybe you swoon over sweets and pasta, or maybe you don't. The point is *not* how much you crave these particular foods, but rather *how your body reacts to them*.

What seems to happen is that carbohydrates, even in small amounts, keep C-Profile people from burning their body fat as fuel.

Jean-Pierre Flatt, Ph.D., a leading researcher in energy metabolism and body-weight reduction at the Department of Biochemistry at the University of Massachusetts Medical School, has shown how this occurs. It has been a long-held belief among scientists that the body readily transforms carbohydrates into fat, which it then stores to use as fuel. Flatt has demonstrated that, to the contrary, excess carbohydrates are not easily converted to fat, but instead are stored as glycogen, a substance the body burns in preference to fat.

In an interview for the newsletter *Obesity Research Update,* Dr. Flatt was asked, "Are carbohydrates important to weight control?" Dr. Flatt responded, "Yes. Carbohydrates determine the amount of fat that is burned. The more carbohydrates you eat, the less fat you burn. The less carbohydrates you eat, the more fat you burn. A person can burn 150–250 grams of fat per day if carbohydrate intake is restricted to 50 grams or less. This is roughly one-third to one-half a pound of fat per day."

So we know that the presence of glycogen in the body will turn down the controller in your brain that tells you to burn fat as if it were a dimmer switch. What we don't know is why, in some people, a small amount of glycogen suddenly signals the switch to turn off altogether.

TREATMENT

I start my patients for the first two weeks on a very restricted carbohydrate intake, just to see what kind of response I get. If a patient loses 5 to 10 pounds over this period, I have my confirmation that carbohydrate sensitivity is the problem.

Essentially, meals during this time consist of nothing but eggs, bacon, meats, poultry, seafood, diet drinks, cheese, cream, nuts, broccoli, cauliflower, and salads. If the approach proves successful, the person can slowly increase his or her carbohydrate intake until he or she is consuming 30–50 grams per day.

Presuming the person continues to do well, I'll keep him or her at this level and offer a low-carbohydrate menu and recipe book as well as various tasty food and shake supplements. The rest is up to the individual.

If the C-Profile wants to remain thin, he or she will have to follow this regimen religiously for the rest of his or her life. Of course, anyone who has ever tried sticking with a high-protein and very low-carbohydrate diet knows how difficult a challenge it can be. This kind of diet is especially tough on women, who generally tend to like carbohydrate foods more than men do. In fact, Julie might very well find the task impossible. That's why, to quiet her cravings and appetite, it is absolutely necessary for her to continue taking her medicines or natural supplements.

It will also help if Julie allows herself plenty of variety in the foods she eats and rewards herself with an occasional "vacation" from the diet.

Unfortunately, the long-term ramifications of this type of high-protein diet are not clear. There is concern that too much protein may be dangerous to the kidneys, but that concern is based on theory, not research. Some studies do suggest

The Body Resists

Even if you love steak, fish, and chicken, giving up or lowering your daily carbohydrate consumption isn't easy to do. In fact, your body may naturally resist all of your very best efforts. Researchers at Ohio State University's Department of Food Science and Technology presented findings at a May 1998 meeting of the American Society of Nutritional Scientists that suggested that's exactly what your body will do.

In an ingenious experiment, scientists gave 25 male college students a Carnation Instant Breakfast™ every day for three weeks. Here's the catch: Three different types of shakes were given. Some of the men got whole-milk shakes, some got skim, and others got skim with sugar added. Each week, the type of shake each man got was changed. Neither the researchers nor the subjects knew who had which kind of shake at any time.

The results showed that over the long term, no matter how much fat or carbohydrate was added to or subtracted from his breakfast shake, each man would unconsciously compensate at other meals the rest of each day, so that by evening, his totals would always be the same.

The results suggest that, just as there's a set point in the brain that determines body weight, there's also a set point for the amount of carbs and fats each person consumes in his or her daily diet.

that, since early humans were primarily hunters and meat eaters, we should be able to adapt healthfully and naturally to this way of nourishing ourselves, but these studies are far from conclusive.

TO SHAKE OR NOT TO SHAKE

In general, I don't see the point in replacing regular meals with special, designer diet foods such as protein shakes because they quickly become monotonous and people stop using them. In this case of C-Profile people, however, protein drinks can have their place.

Some people get bored with eggs, sausage, and cheese after a while, so drinking a shake now and then actually adds some variety to their meals, which is very appealing. In fact, I've treated a few brave souls who jump-started their new low-carb eating plan by consuming five protein shakes a day for the first two weeks, and after that, one shake before each meal to further curb their appetite.

Shakes can also be useful in getting those last 5 to 10 pounds off—the ones that always seems so difficult to lose.

Obviously, shakes shouldn't be the centerpiece of your diet over the long term. They simply don't offer the nutrition that the human body needs. I would also recommend that anyone temporarily using shakes as a primary food and calorie source take a multivitamin every day.

8

Guess What Doesn't Work!

Check out any pharmacy, supermarket, or health-food store, and you'll find enough weight-loss products, both prescription and over the counter, to make you dizzy. Then there are the various programs, approaches, and devices offered through infomercials, magazines, and alternative practitioners.

So what works and what doesn't? We've already talked about the most effective tools you can use to turn off your hunger switch. Is there any value at all to any of the other "pounds-off" promises the marketplace offers you every day?

Here's what we know about some of them.

ACUPUNCTURE

Most people these days have some passing familiarity with this ancient form of healing from China—or have, at least, heard of it—but few are aware that it may actually be an effective weight-reducing technique.

Acupuncture represents a holistic approach to health, a balancing of all the opposing forces within you. Hair-thin needles are inserted along "meridian points" on the body. Meridians might best be described as where energy can be stopped, diverted, or increased.

To some Western doctors, all this sounds more like poetry than medicine, but there is no doubt that acupuncture has proven effective in the control of both acute and chronic pain. In China it is even used in place of anesthesia during surgery!

There was some initial promise when a study in Taiwan followed 45 subjects with diet, exercise, and acupuncture. They lost an average of 9.7 pounds after 2 months. But obviously, the diet and exercise could have given that modest degree of weight loss over such a short period.

I have had patients tell me that ear acupuncture makes mildly spicy foods tastier. But I have never seen acupuncture cause weight loss, and some controlled clinical trials have all proved negative.

In all fairness, I have seen remarkable improvements in pain relief and control of anxiety. It is therefore conceivable that combined with medications, acupuncture could control stress eating in conjunction with the drugs. This study has not been done and maybe should be. Multiapproach therapy is almost always preferable to the single approach. So acupuncture could still be useful as part of a multimodality treatment of obesity. Forget it, though, as the sole regimen.

AMPHETAMINES

Forty years ago, these drugs represented the gold standard for weight-loss medications. They are powerful appetite inhibitors, but they are also dangerous and addicting. People who use them over an extended period of time often become restless and nervous. Many develop the "shakes," a chronic and noticeable trembling of the hands. Insomnia is common. Overdoses can cause depression, psychosis, and death. Enough said?

AROMATHERAPY

This treatment is based on using the essential oils of certain plants. These oils are inhaled, diluted, or added to a bath. The inhaler is the most convenient form and is prepared by mixing 15 drops of bergamof oil and 10 drops of fennel oil in a small airtight container. The oils are mixed very gently and then used as an inhalant for hunger control.

Dr. Alan Hirsch has done most of the research on this therapy. He studied 3,000 subjects who inhaled green apple, peppermint, and banana odors whenever they experienced hunger or cravings. Those who responded best were medium- to large-frame people and were chocolate cravers. The subjects lost an average of 1 pound per week over six months. It is theorized that the odors work directly on the appetite center of the brain. People who suffer with asthma or migraine headaches shouldn't use these inhalers.

I've never tried this form of treatment, so I can't comment on it fairly. There seems to be some promise here for certain individuals. The weight loss is slow but reasonable. It doesn't work for everyone, and it's likely that a tolerance would develop over time. Again, I wouldn't suggest using it by itself, but rather alongside other approaches.

CHROMIUM

You've seen the ads; you've heard the claims:

- "Lose the fat, keep the muscle."
- "Lose unwanted fat while reshaping your body to a leaner, trimmer, firmer physique."
- "Improves your metabolism so your body relies more on using stored fat and less on proteins . . . resulting in more muscle and less fat."
- "No dieting, no exercise required."
- "Melts the fat away."
- "Plays a key role in reducing fat through better appetite control and increased metabolic rate."
- "Dramatically reduces body fat, lowers cholesterol, builds leaner muscle mass."
- "Works by making your body more sensitive to the hormone insulin."

If all, or even some of these claims are true, then chromium must be a candidate for weight-loss miracle of the century.

Chemically, chromium is a trace mineral, a substance that exists naturally in the human body in minute amounts. It's certainly necessary for good health, but should we encourage people to use large doses in supplement form? Is it safe and effective?

I first became interested in chromium when another physician called to confer with me about one of his patients who had come to me for help with weight control. The physician said he was impressed with the results his patient had achieved on our program, and wondered if we had ever used chromium as a natural appetite suppressant. He had used it for years to better control blood-sugar levels in diabetic patients, and he claimed it also helped them lose weight.

I try to be open minded to new approaches to weight control, and I am normally very receptive to the idea that vitamin and mineral supplements can have great benefits for the human body. I take daily megadoses of antioxidant vitamins every morning to help prevent cancer and heart disease. I even believe alternative therapies make sense in the management of some patients.

When I heard that chromium might help some of my patients, I immediately began collecting all of the literature on chromium that I could find.

The theory went like this: Chromium transports sugars and amino acids, which are the building blocks of proteins and muscle, into the cells of the body. Therefore, if you take lots of chromium, you will build lots of muscle, which will then burn lots of fat for fuel. I immediately became suspicious. The "more is better" theory hardly ever proves true where the human body is concerned. It's like saying that if a little fat in your diet is necessary and good for you, lots and lots of fat must be even better.

Most of the early work on chromium was done by Gary Evans, a chemist who works in the nutrition field. He developed a process to synthetically manufacture chromium picolinate and did two field studies on weight training.

In the first, he gave 200 mcg of chromium picolinate each day to a group of college students who were training with weights. He reported that after six weeks, the students showed an average 3.5-pound increase in muscle mass, while a control group taking a placebo showed slightly less than a pound of increase per subject.

The second study, carried out on college football players, used the same method and, according to Evans, yielded similar results.

Criticism of the studies has been vehement. Hank Lukaski, Research Leader at the United States Department of Agriculture Human Nutrition Research Center stated in April 1994 at the North Dakota Academy of Science, "For young men trying to maximize their strength—or anyone else—chromium picolinate has no effect on building muscle, reducing body fat, changing body composition, decreasing weight, or increasing strength."

Robert LeFavi and colleagues, in the *International Journal of Sport Nutrition*, have criticized Evans's scientific method and questioned both the effectiveness and safety of chromium supplements.

Unfortunately, only a few studies other than Evans's have been done. In one, football players from the University of Massachusetts showed no change in body composition after nine weeks of taking chromium supplements and doing intense conditioning exercises every day. In another study, 35 healthy men reported the same results after eight weeks of chromium use, although researchers did note that the subjects were excreting five times the normal amount of chromium in their urine.

A study in 1996 showed slightly more positive results. People taking 200–400 mcg of chromium per day showed an

Let the Buyer Beware

Here are some of the weight-loss scams and frauds that the Federal Trade Commission is warning consumers against:

- Any program that promises you'll lose 30 pounds in 30 days

- Skin patches

- Shoe insoles

- Fat blockers that purport to prevent fat absorption (with the exception of Orlistat)

- Fat "magnets" that purport to flush fat out of the body before absorption

- Diet teas

- Products containing glucomannan, chromium picolinate, hydroxycitrate, guar gum, fat emulsifiers, cellulose/fiber, and ox bile extracts

- Fiber tablets

- Bee pollen

- Laxatives

- Electrical muscle stimulators

- Passive-motion exercise devices

- Hunger-suppressing ear cuffs

- Acupuncture devices

- Body wrappings, belts, or girdles

- Any of the 111 over-the-counter substances the FDA has declared not safe or effective for weight loss average loss of 4.2 pounds of fat over two and a half months. If these results actually show what chromium can do, there doesn't seem to be much cause for celebration.

FIBER

Chromium isn't the only over-the-counter substance currently marketed as a miracle cure for obesity. Products containing high amounts of bulk fiber have also enjoyed a lot of fanfare. They're supposed to fill you up and, because fiber isn't stored or metabolized by the body, you don't gain any weight. Cellulose and other food fibers actually will make you feel more full, but the effect is only temporary. Soon you'll find yourself facing the old cravings again. By the way, there is no evidence to support the claim that fiber stops the body from absorbing fat, or that it speeds up metabolism. It's all hype that exploits the desperation of people who are in genuine need.

Although neither chromium nor fiber seems to be of much help in losing weight, other "natural" substances and approaches have shown promising results.

CHITOSAN®

Chiten is the fiber found in the outer shells of soft-shelled fish, such as shrimp and lobster, and insects. Recently, it has been used in the manufacture of a fiber supplement, Chitosan®, and touted as a weight-loss product.

The manufacturer's claim is that Chitosan® will absorb twelve times its own weight in fat from the food you eat and pass through the body undigested, taking the unwanted fat with it.

I've seen no substantial evidence to support this claim. Animal studies show minor positive effects from the product. It does seem to lower fat absorption slightly, by about 8 percent, and works better when supplemented with vitamin C; but it also lowers protein and calcium absorption. If you take this product, be prepared to boost your calcium and protein intake in your diet or with supplements.

No study has shown this product to have any effect on weight loss, and the cost may be prohibitive.

CITRIMAX

For centuries people in Asia have used an extract from an evergreen plant, called the Malabar tamarind, to season their food. The extract has a sweet, acid taste, and seems to make people who use it feel more full and satisfied after a meal. The scientific name for the extract is hydroxy citric acid (HCA). It is marketed in this country under the name Citrimax.

Theoretically, HCA works by diverting carbohydrates and fats into the liver for storage as a substance called glycogen, rather than into cells for fat storage.

It was promoted as an appetite suppressant and cholesterol reducer. There was some initial enthusiasm and hope for this product, but it has been a dismal failure when put to the test in clinical trials.

A study in 1998 at St. Luke's/Roosevelt Hospital in New York showed HCA ineffective at causing weight loss in humans at the standard dose of 1,500 mg per day. The group taking the placebo actually lost more weight than those on the HCA did!

In August 1999, results of another very well-designed study from the University of Colorado showed that HCA does not cause fat or calorie burning.

Another study, reported in June 1997, was done on 50 overweight women, who showed no significant weight loss after six weeks. These people took chromium as well as caffeine.

More significantly, studies done on animals by the drug manufacturer Hoffmann-La Roche showed that HCA caused testicular atrophy. The company didn't dare proceed to human studies.

In summary, the product is ineffective and, if you're a male, possibly even hazardous to your health. I'd avoid it!

ESSENTIAL FATTY ACIDS

While it's true that too much dietary fat can be dangerous, it's also true that you need to eat some fat to be healthy.

Essential fatty acids (EFAs) are fats that come from plants and fish. They come in two varieties: omega-6 (linolenic acid) and omega-3 (linoleic acid). You get plenty of omega-6 in the vegetable oils you use when you cook, make salads, and bake. Omega-3 isn't so plentiful. You find it only in fish oil and oils made from canola, soy, and flax.

For good health, you need to consume about three times as much omega-6 as you do omega-3. If you go on a very low-fat diet and don't get enough of these nutrients, your skin will eventually become very dry and your hair will start to fall out. It takes a while, sometimes two to three months, for these effects to appear because your body stores

EFAs in plentiful amounts, and it takes you some time to use them up.

In extreme cases, a patient deficient in EFAs will form gallstones, a very serious condition. If there is no fat whatsoever in the diet, a person will die within two weeks. So whenever you're on a diet, it's a good idea to supplement EFAs.

On the plus side, some recent evidence shows that EFAs can enhance fat burning and increase metabolism. They can also lower cholesterol levels and raise calcium levels in the body.

I supplement my patients with 1,300 mg of oil of evening primrose twice per day. I also suggest they take one 1,000-mg capsule of flax oil every day. This combination gives them plenty of omega-6 and omega-3 oils in the proper ratio, and eliminates any of the harmful side effects associated with low-fat diets.

HYPNOSIS

Hypnosis is another popular alternative for weight control. I've had a few patients swear by it. Unfortunately, even when it works, the results are temporary at best.

The general idea of hypnosis is to induce a mental and physical state of relaxation through suggestion, which will then allow you to gain better control of your eating behavior.

In those for whom it's successful, the relaxation phase is the result of a rise in brain-serotonin levels. It's very much like taking a low dose of a serotonin-raising drug. Both approaches can lead to less compulsive eating, but in both cases, the results are only temporary unless combined with a norepinephrine agent, like phentermine or ephedra/caffeine. Remember, if only your serotonin level increases, you'll eventually *gain* weight.

Hypnosis may be valuable when combined with either natural or pharmacological agents to give an even greater serotonin balance, which would, in theory, lead to better control of cravings, compulsive eating, and binges. However, this combination effect has never been studied.

HERBS

Herbalists have recommended all kinds of plant therapies to help people lose weight. Unfortunately, most don't work. The following popular herbs seem to have little or no positive weight-loss effects, either among my own patients or in any of the clinical trials I've examined: St. John's wort, kelp, gotu kola, ginkgo, garcinia, parsley, dandelion, corn silk, juniper berries, seaweed, chickweed, fennel, and ginseng.

ORLISTAT

This drug, sold commercially as Xenical®, keeps you from absorbing much of the fat from the food you eat. Clinical trials show that people have lost 10 percent of their body weight with regular use. Among my patients, however, the side effects of the drug—which include greasy diarrhea, cramping, fecal incontinence, and oily discharge—were so severe that I stopped recommending its use. Whatever happened in the clinical trials, I've never known anyone who tolerates using the stuff long enough for it to be effective.

SLIM FAST™

This is a low-calorie meal replacement milkshake that actually seems to work for some people. However, it has two drawbacks. First, it contains 40 grams of carbohydrates and 35 grams of sugar, making it a disaster for people with a C-Profile. Second, while many people find the taste pleasant, drinking it every day can become extremely monotonous, and the overall low-calorie diet of which it is a part is very hard to comply with for longer than a few weeks.

9

The Uncooperative Doctor

So, you are seriously overweight, you have not been able to lose weight by conventional methods, and you want to turn back the thermostat in your brain. You could use all-natural supplements, of course, but you don't feel comfortable taking anything, even over-the-counter agents, for any length of time without medical supervision. Besides, you have a suspicion that prescription medication might work better and faster.

I recommend you always consult a physician before you embark on any of the regimens I've previously described. But what if your family doctor refuses even to consider starting you on a program that includes weight-loss medications or supplements? Or your doctor does not feel competent to manage such a program? Or you do not currently have a doctor?

If any of these cases describe your situation, it may be time to begin searching for someone who can help you. You need to find someone who can comfort and console you, as well as counsel and medicate you for the treatment of your condition.

For many years, bariatricians—physicians who specialized in treating overweight patients—were referred to simply as "diet doctors." They were usually looked down upon and mistrusted by the larger medical community, and perhaps with good reason. After all, almost nothing these doctors tried worked permanently, and patients could end up handing over a fortune in medical bills by the time they realized they were spinning their wheels.

It is only recently that bariatrics came into its own as a serious branch of science. These days, the average bariatrician is a knowledgeable specialist who has attended many courses and seminars after completing training in some other speciality, such as internal medicine. He or she is well equipped to manage the problem of obesity in the general population.

If your family physician can refer you to a qualified bariatrician, your problem is solved. If not, you can contact the American Society of Bariatric Physicians for a list of addresses and phone numbers of bariatric physicians. The society also offers valuable tapes on weight loss and related subjects. Write to The American Society of Bariatric Physicians, 5600 S. Quebec Street, Suite 109A, Englewood, CO 80111. You can also e-mail the society at bariatric@asbp.org, or check out its Web site at www.asbp.org.

A list of weight-loss doctors is also given in Appendix C.

KNOW THE SIGNS

There are some clues to look for in your search to make sure you are putting yourself in the hands of someone who knows what he or she is doing.

The Diet Mill

This is the medical office in which one doctor will examine as many as 80 patients per day. Each appointment consists of a 5-minute visit, which may or may not be with a qualified professional, in which pills, shots, or liquid medication, and—if you're lucky—some brief counseling are given. The come-on here is the price, which is usually irresistibly low. I can only advise you to remember that you get what you pay for. If prices seem unbelievably low, you can bet you're dealing with a very high-volume business that will neither view nor treat you with concern, care, or respect.

Shots

If a doctor starts talking needles to help you shed pounds, say, "No, thank you," and leave. I can think of no diet medication that needs to be injected. Usually, instead of real medication, you are getting a dose of B vitamins, which do nothing to help you lose weight. If you have a vitamin deficiency, by all means, take all the vitamins you need, either by changing your diet or by going to your local health-food store and buying some pills. A poor diet can indeed result in beriberi, anemia, or a host of other conditions, but none of this has anything to do with losing weight.

The fact is that, to many patients, shots seem like magic. If it comes in a hypodermic syringe, it looks mysterious, potent, really "medical." When you're taking medicine, however, you need to take some control over your own safety. You can't tell what's in a syringe, or how high the concentration is. It doesn't come with a label.

Again, some medicines must be given by injection, but those used for weight loss do not. If your only medical problem is that you're overweight, you don't need shots.

Overdosing

Even if a doctor gives you plenty of his or her time, doesn't offer any shots, and seems to know about weight-loss medications and supplements, it is absolutely essential that he or she prescribe these agents in low doses. One of the most important aspects of the breakthrough in this field is that, in combination, medications can be administered at minimal dosages, which means their chances for causing side effects are greatly reduced. This is not to say there are no exceptions to the rule. Sometimes we have to prescribe standard or higher doses, but only in very rare circumstances. Unless a doctor can give you some specific reasons for prescribing higher doses in your particular case, find someone else who will be more prudent and more concerned with the health of his or her patients.

THE GOOD GUYS

Now that you know who *not* to go to, let's take a look at some of the qualities you'll want in the person to whom you *do* go.

A Realistic Medical Philosophy

First and foremost, the doctor must understand and be willing to treat obesity as the illness that it is, not as a psychological or character problem that can be solved by willpower alone. You can get that kind of nonsense from any commercial weight-loss center; you don't need to go to a doctor for it. The doctor must understand that obesity is both serious and complex, that is, a result of many factors, including heredity and brain chemistry. The doctor must also be willing to treat you as a chronic, long-term patient because, as we have seen, being overweight is a life-long problem.

All this comes down to the general philosophy of the doctor. Call ahead and ask about the general approach, with regard to weight loss, of any program or physician you're interested in. Remember, you and your doctor will be working together for a long time. It should be a happy partnership.

Board Certification

You may also want to ask if the physician you're considering is board certified in his or her field. Although this does not necessarily ensure competence, it does guarantee that the doctor has passed a very rigorous examination in his or her specialty, and that even to take that exam, he or she first had to complete internship and residency requirements. Again, certification is no guarantee you'll get a good doctor, but lack of certification should be a red flag. Think about the way you would choose an accountant. If he's got a degree and is a CPA, he may or may not be competent, but if he has neither, it's a pretty safe bet that you don't want him filling out your income tax forms for the IRS.

Appropriate Training

Find out where the doctor received his or her medical training. Did he or she graduate from a medical school and residency

Good News from the IRS

You wouldn't think that IRS policy has much to do with weight loss, but in fact it does. How? By giving you a tax break for getting into a weight-loss program. Recently, and for the first time, the IRS has said that it will allow taxpayers who itemize their returns to deduct the cost of weight-loss programs as a medical expense. Covered areas include medical counseling, nutritional counseling, drugs, and surgery. Items not covered include health-club dues and, unfortunately, nutritional supplements. Also, the program needs to be undertaken at a physician's direction, and it must treat an existing disease, such as diabetes, through weight loss. Programs undertaken simply for general good health can't be deducted. Remember, medical expenses must be greater than 7.5 percent of your adjusted gross income before you can deduct them.

program that are affiliated with a university? Community hospital residency programs often produce some very fine doctors, but sometimes their standards are not so high or so rigorously enforced as those held by university hospitals. This is a small point, but if you're comparing physicians, all else being equal, you're probably better off going to someone who is university trained.

Clinical Background

Make sure the doctor you're considering has plenty of clinical experience working with all of the illnesses associated with obesity, including hypertension, diabetes, heart disease, and lipid abnormalities. The doctor should also be alert to the increased vulnerability to other diseases, including various cancers, joint problems, and gallbladder disease. In short, his or her background should be in primary care rather than in a specialty such as ophthalmology, dermatology, or psychiatry. Internists, gynecologists, and practitioners of family medicine all represent much better choices, as obesity-related health problems tend to show up far more often in the offices of these doctors.

Finally, when you consider going to any physician for help in weight control, ask if he or she is a registered member of the American Society of Bariatric Physicians and has submitted to its carefully developed standards of care.

10

Keeping the Switch in the Off Position

Many, if not most, people who take these medications immediately begin looking forward to the day they can stop taking them. As soon as they get their weight down to a normal level, they think they will be "cured" and they can stop taking pills.

I wish it were so, but for most patients, unfortunately, it is not. True, a few lucky individuals will find they can maintain healthy eating habits even after they've gone off their medications, but most will require very low maintenance doses for the rest of their lives.

DON'T TAKE IT PERSONALLY

Once again, it is important to remember that being over-weight is a chronic, medical condition, *not* a character flaw. I would not expect a patient with elevated cholesterol to show normal lipid levels in her blood if she stopped her medications; neither would I expect healthy blood-sugar levels in a severely diabetic person who suddenly discontinued his insulin shots. In the same way, I don't expect most obese patients who go off their Hunger Switch program to continue enjoying freedom from food obsessions.

It is the word "freedom" that makes most people confused. How can you be free if you're dependent upon medications?

Where your weight is concerned, the answer is simple. You can use weight-control agents to help free you from overeating, or you can continue to overeat and be free from the use of weight-control agents. It's sort of like saying you can work to free yourself from poverty, or you can remain poor to free yourself from the need to work. The choice is yours.

A HORSE OF A DIFFERENT COLOR

Most people don't realize that losing weight and maintaining the lost weight are two very different animals. Losing weight requires an adjustment of brain chemistry, which leads to an adjustment of the brain thermostat controlling your weight. Once the body reaches its new setting, your weight will level off and won't go any lower.

Why? The brain is always in full control of where it wants your weight to be. The final number has nothing to do with ideal body weights, insurance company charts, or BMI indices. Your brain doesn't care about charts. It only cares about balancing its own chemistry.

THIS IS HOW WE DO IT

Compared to losing weight, maintenance is somewhat easier, but it requires a serious, long-term commitment. Your job now is simple: Keep your brain chemistry in proper balance forever.

You may find that you can stop pills and maintain your weight for six months to even two years. But at some point, your brain's chemistry will start to go out of balance again, and your weight will begin to make its way upward.

It's a frustrating situation because it will happen without your changing your eating habits. You can try to eat even less, but your weight will continue to climb. It may even exceed your initial weight. The reason for this is clear. Your brain chemistry is in full control, and it's telling you to store energy in the form of fat rather than burn it as fuel. Diet and exercise can't keep up with the new situation and inevitably fail.

So you have to keep taking the pills, just as if you were treating any other chronic medical condition such as hypertension, elevated cholesterol, diabetes, or depression. There is no cure, only control. The pills will control your brain chemistry, which will in turn control your weight. Only genetic engineering or manipulation will cure weight problems.

Fortunately, the average person can maintain his or her new weight by taking medications or supplements on Monday, Wednesday, and Friday only. If that doesn't work, try taking them every day, but cut the dose in half. It's that simple.

Nature's Fat Fighter

Two recent studies, one published in the December 2000 issue of the *Journal of Nutrition*, and the other presented at a meeting of The American Chemical Society in Washington, D.C. in August 2000, both confirm the fat-fighting effects of a substance that occurs naturally in meat, poultry, and dairy products called CLA (conjugated linoleic acid). About 3 grams of the stuff daily (1 gram before each meal), along with very light exercise, safely and effectively reduced the amount of fat people carried in their bodies, while increasing the amount of muscle. When people were maintaining their weight, CLA helped to make sure that any pounds they gained back came in the form of muscle. So if you're determined to go off your medications or supplements, you might consider taking 1 gram of CLA with each meal, every day.

EXERCISE CAN PLAY A ROLE

Although exercising doesn't do much to help you lose weight, it can have some value in maintenance. It will help to raise your metabolism and burn off any extra calories you may consume. However, exercise alone won't keep you at your ideal weight.

The problem is that the exercise has to be very strenuous, regular, and long term if it's to carry the burden of your entire weight-maintenance. In the absence of medications, you would have to work out one to two hours every single day for life. Most people can't commit themselves to a lifetime of exercising on those terms. Sooner or later, circumstances interfere with almost any exercise program. It's a fact of life, and there is no point in preaching otherwise.

MAINTAINING WITH A HIGH-MAINTENANCE DOCTOR

As difficult as it might be for you to accept that you may have to take weight-controlling medications or supplements for the rest of your life, it will probably prove even more difficult for your doctor to accept.

Any physician who is unfamiliar with these drugs will balk at the idea of your taking prescription medications on a long-term basis. When you ask the doctor why, you'll hear the same old arguments you thought had been thrown out with last year's garbage: Obesity isn't a medical problem; obesity isn't serious enough to treat with drugs; weight-loss medications lead to addiction; etc., etc., etc.

It's disheartening, but be patient. Remember, you're thinking "helpful medications," but the doctor's thinking "dangerous drugs." I've been through this with my own patients, so I know how the doctor feels. It's one thing to agree in theory that a drug is safe. It is altogether another to prescribe it, long term, for a patient. The doctor may not be able to shake his or her recollections of amphetamine abuse in the 1960s. He or she may be recalling the indiscriminate use of thalidamide, which led to birth defects, or the overprescribing of Valium® for anxiety, which turned a large number of unsuspecting people into addicts. Or the doctor may have swallowed all the recent propaganda about ephedra.

The best you can do is try to talk rationally with your doctor about his or her concerns. If they apply to your particular health condition, listen to your doctor. If, on the other hand, they have more to do with his or her general philosophy of drug or nutritional therapy, the doctor may be willing to reconsider his or her position in the light of any information you can give. Below are some items that might come up for discussion.

1. *Obesity may be chronic and result from genetic or physiological factors, but it isn't truly a medical condition.*

Remind your doctor gently that obesity is, in fact, more a "medical" condition than is high blood pressure. It has a stronger genetic link; displays more symptoms, including fatigue, joint pain, and shortness of breath upon minimal exertion; and often leads to depression. It also carries more greater social consequences than do many conditions generally accepted as "medical."

Perhaps it would be more appropriate to compare obesity to diabetes. Both are inherited; both are associated with other, complicating health problems; and both can be medically controlled.

Actually, most illnesses that confront physicians would fit easily into the same category. With the exception of non-viral infectious diseases, most are chronic, incurable, and to some degree controllable. Think about it: heart failure, cardiac rhythm disturbances, angina, emphysema, chronic bronchitis, asthma, sickle cell anemia, migraine headaches, genital herpes, lipid abnormalities, allergies, arthritis . . . the list goes on.

Most of these conditions are treated with medications that can have grave side effects. Unfortunately, diet drugs and supplements seem held to a higher standard than are drugs for other diseases.

2. *Obesity isn't a serious enough problem to justify any approach other than diet and exercise.*

This one is easy. We've already been through the statistics, but just to recount them in brief, you can remind your doctor that obesity doubles your risk for hypertension, heart attack, gallbladder disease, stroke, diabetes, and premature death. It also increases your chance of getting cancer of the uterus, ovary, prostate, and colon. Breast-cancer risk goes up 50 percent in women over the age of thirty if they are a mere 20 pounds overweight.

Then there are the psychological and social problems. Overweight people suffer from discrimination, prejudice, and contempt in nearly every area of their lives. Not only does it wreck their self-esteem and hurl them into depression, but it affects them economically as well.

3. *Long-term treatment with pills, whether they're prescribed or over -the-counter, is dangerous and addictive.*

The data doesn't support this idea. Furthermore, these substances are not new. Many have been on the market and in use for thirty years, and nowhere do we find, in all that time, a slew of doctors complaining about addiction as a side effect.

4. *Long-term treatment isn't generally accepted by the medical community.*

True enough, and it will probably take another five or ten years before it is. In the meantime, no doctor wants to be thought of as a quack, or even as someone practicing on the fringe of accepted medical procedure. The medical establishment moves slowly. I know this from personal experience.

What About Vitamins?

Many people ask me about supplemental vitamins and/or minerals as a part of an overall healthy eating pattern for life. Multivitamins are not very useful in my opinion. They give too little of each nutrient to be beneficial.

I prefer my patients to take significant amounts of individual nutrients. For prevention of heart disease, I recommend 400–800 mcg of folic acid per day and a mixed Tocopherol vitamin E at 400–800 IU per day. Selenium 200 mcg is an excellent choice for cancer prevention. Several studies have shown a decrease in cancer risk by about 60 percent when taking selenium. If you want B vitamins, then get a high-potency B complex with at least 100 mg of each B vitamin.

Some patients have told me that horse chestnut is excellent for fluid retention and edema and black cohosh and soy isoflavones are both very good for hot flashes, which occur during postmenopause.

In the mid 1980s, when I first left my residency in internal medicine to open a private practice, there were only whispers about the significance of elevated cholesterol levels. Treating them with medication was absolutely taboo. Diet and exercise were universally prescribed, except in the most severe cases. Then the famous Framingham Study announced its data, which revealed a 2-percent increase in the risk for heart attack with every 1-percent increase in blood cholesterol level.

Suddenly, everyone rushed to get their arms punctured and their blood checked. Everywhere you went, from the office to dinner parties, you heard people talking about it.

When a pharmaceutical company released a cholesterol-lowering drug called Mevacor®, physicians began prescribing it as if it were a miracle in a bottle. It didn't take long for other companies to jump on the bandwagon. Soon, other cholesterol-lowering drugs crowded onto the market. Overnight the idea of using medications to treat high blood cholesterol became as widely accepted as treating headaches with aspirin.

We're not there yet with weight-controlling drugs or supplements, but we may not be so far away as you might think. A headline in the July 20, 1994 *Wall Street Journal* read, "Respect for Diet Pills Rises as Studies Shed New Light on Obesity. FDA Considers Brain Drugs to Lift Mood and Ease Compulsion to Overeat." The article goes on, ". . . This new view is sweeping through medical circles. . . . Doctors are already treating thousands of patients according to the new neuroscientific approach, using older drugs. As their ranks swell, they pose a serious threat to the two-billion-dollar industry that sells weight-loss programs based on using diet and exercise to shed pounds. Dieters generally gain back most of their weight within three to five years."

5. *As with many weight-loss agents, these will become ineffective over time as a patient's body develops tolerance to them.*

Dr. Albert Stunkard, a professor at the University of Pennsylvania School of Medicine, thoroughly addressed this issue in a lecture on the subject:

105

For many years it has been established practice to pre-scribe appetite suppressant medications for only limited periods of time. The evidence for this belief is obscure, and a set point interpretation of tolerance makes clear its limitations. In terms of body weight, tolerance to appetite suppressants does not develop, which means that the old argument against use—the loss of effi-ciency—is no longer valid. These agents retain their efficiency. Paradoxically, it is precisely this maintenance of efficiency that argues against their short-term use. If any benefits of appetite suppressants are lost when the medications are discontinued, then such medication should not be used on a short-term basis. Current policy appears to be diametrically opposed to national use of appetite suppressant medication, and current practice appears wholly unwarranted. Furthermore, the myth of tolerance seems to have prevented use of appetite sup-pressants in precisely those situations in which they are indicated—over the long term.

Physicians tend to be a skeptical bunch, myself included. But with a little patience, time, and effort, you may well be able to educate your doctor on the advantages of the new medical approach to weight control. It's certainly worth a try.

11.

Choosing a Healthful Diet

If you want to be healthy, you need to eat a healthful diet and do some form of exercise on a regular basis. It's the human condition. No pill can change it.

Now before you start groaning, let me explain what's meant by a "healthful" diet. It does not mean you have to reduce the number of calories you eat. This is not about weight loss. It's about eating foods that will keep you well and avoiding ones that can do you harm. There's no point to losing weight if you're just going to end up being sickly.

So what makes a healthful diet? The answer won't surprise you: a diet low in fat. Why?

According to the *Journal of the American Medical Association*, 300,000 people a year die from diseases associ-

ated with a high-fat diet, including heart disease, high blood pressure, stroke, cancer, arthritis, and multiple sclerosis.

CHOOSING HEALTHFUL FOODS

Although you should be eating a low-fat diet, a little fat in your meals is necessary for sustenance. So it isn't necessary to go crazy looking for foods that contain practically no fat at all. Instead, look at the nutritional labels on the foods you buy, then plug the numbers you find into the following formula, which was devised by a nutritionist:

Protein (in grams) + carbohydrate (in grams) = A
Fat (in grams) × 5 = B

If A is larger than B, it's a healthy food. If B is larger, however, perhaps you should save this food for special occasions.

Let's see how this works for two popular snacks: potato chips and pretzels.

- Potato chips have 9 grams of fat, 2 grams of protein, and 14 grams of carbohydrates.

  2 (protein) + 14 (carbohydrate) = 16 (A)
  9 (fat) × 5 = 45 (B)

  A is smaller than B, so potato chips are a fatty food.

- Pretzels have 0 grams of fat, 1 gram of protein, and 19 grams of carbohydrates.

  1 (protein) + 19 (carbohydrate) = 20 (A)
  0 (fat) × 5 = 0 (B)

  A is larger than B, so pretzels are a healthy food.

Why Calorie-Restricting Diets Don't Work

Research clearly shows that the number of calories you eat every day doesn't have very much to do with your weight. The HANES I Survey of 1971–1975, for example, looked at the calorie intake and energy expenditure of over 20,000 Americans and discovered that thin people, on average, actually eat more calories than obese people. Other studies have reached similar conclusions.

Martha, one of my patients, is a typical case. She had been on one diet or another ever since she had been a teenager. All of the diets forced her to keep her calorie intake down to the 500–1,000 calorie-per-day range. Not a nice way to live, but it did cause her to lose weight, on average about 40 pounds over three months. The problem was that after six months, she would gain back 45–50 pounds. After the cycle had repeated itself again and again, it became clear that not only had dieting failed to make Martha lose weight, it had actually caused her to gain some. Martha's story is a common one, and it's an object lesson for all of us: Losing weight is not about having the willpower to restrict calories.

For those who don't want to do all the math, the simpler method is to locate "total fat per serving" on the nutrition labels of all the foods you eat in a day, add up the numbers, and try to keep the total at about 20 grams.

But for heaven's sake, don't worry if you occasionally dine out at a restaurant or grab a meal at a fast-food place, where you don't know how much fat you're eating. If you set a bunch of rules for yourself that make you feel miserable and deprived, you won't follow them for long. Remember, you're creating a new, healthy lifestyle, not a program that will only last for a few weeks or months. Make rules you can follow, and don't beat yourself over the head if you break them once in a while.

For example, if you find yourself eating at restaurants on a regular basis, just be reasonable with your choices. Use common sense. Check the menu or ask the server for low-fat selections. Grilled and skinless chicken breast, baked or broiled fish, pork loin, and even shrimp, lobster, and crab are delicious and healthy.

I remember the look of shock on the face of one of my patients, a young woman named Judy, when she told me that she still found herself wishing for chocolate cake on certain days. My advice to her? Eat chocolate cake. She immediately protested that she had always been warned to avoid this particular pleasure at all cost. If she had "always been warned," then chocolate cake must have always presented her with an unusually strong temptation. I asked her if she thought she could live the rest of her life without it. She sheepishly admitted that she couldn't imagine such a life. "Then why set yourself up to fail?" I asked her. "Eat the cake."

She still looked unsure. She wasn't so much concerned about her health. She was concerned about her weight. She was afraid that one taste of her favorite food would lead to a binge. I reminded her that as long as she was following the program for her profile and her hunger switch was in the "off" position, bingeing wouldn't become a problem.

Rules for Dining Out

Here are some easy-to-follow suggestions for choosing healthy fare from restaurant menus:

- Choose vegetables and whole grains rather than fish; fish rather than chicken; and chicken rather than beef or pork.

- Avoid sauces made with cream, butter, or cheese. These include Alfredo, au gratin, and bearnaise sauces.

- Go for grilled, broiled, poached, or steamed foods rather than fried and sauteed.

- Choose whole-grain breads, pastas, and rice rather than their white counterparts.

- Stop eating when you're no longer hungry. Wrap the rest in a doggie bag.

- Choose marinara instead of bolognese sauce in Italian restaurants.

- Use oil and vinegar instead of creamier salad dressings, such as Thousand Island.

- Choose fruit-based desserts rather than chocolate; sorbet rather ice cream; and flan rather than crème brulee.

It is precisely in this kind of situation—an uncontrollable craving for carbohydrates—that brain-chemistry balancing agents do their best work. I knew that after eating a small slice of cake, she would feel satisfied and lose her craving, and I told her so. Nor would she be bothered by obsessive thoughts about food—any food!

I now have a patient who loves to go around telling people that she "has her cake and eats it too." Ah, well. I suppose eating less corn doesn't necessarily make you less corny.

RULES TO EAT BY

Here are some general guidelines I give to my patients to help them make sensible, healthy eating choices.

Eat Lean, Protein-Rich Foods

These include low-fat dairy products, such as skim milk, low-fat yogurt, and egg whites; all seafood, including shrimp, crab, and lobster; lean cuts of meat, such as pork loin and ground sirloin; and beans.

Eat Any Vegetable

Whether fresh, frozen, or canned; broccoli, cauliflower, peas, corn, kale, asparagus, and yams are all good choices. The only exception is avocado, which is high in fat.

Eat Any Fruit

Be careful of fruit juices, however, which can be full of sugar, both natural and added.

Eat Whole-Grain Foods

These include whole wheat, bulgur wheat, couscous, and whole-grain breads.

Go Easy on White and Refined Foods

Especially avoid anything that has refined sugar or refined white flour in it, including so-called "low fat" products, which are full of sugar. They'll raise your insulin level, and if you have a C-Profile, pack on pounds. They'll also raise levels of a group of blood fats called triglycerides. Too much of these blood fats can raise your risk for heart disease.

Eat with Common Sense

What about eating out at the homes of friends, or at dinner parties, or worst of all, at wedding receptions, birthday parties, and anniversary celebrations? If the food choices available are limited, or if you find yourself facing a huge pile of food dolloped out by an overly generous caterer in the serving line, eat only a portion of it. I know, you're thinking that when you were a child, your parents ordered you to "clean your plate, down to the very last crumb" in a misguided effort to look out for your nutrition. Perhaps some teacher may have advised you to remember the poor, starving children in some third-world country whenever you were tempted to "waste" good food. Well, you're no longer a child, and you need not follow bad advice from people with good intentions.

Some of you may have tried most of these dietary recommendations in the past, but failed to follow them for any length of time. If you're on track with your profile plan, you won't fail this time. Why? Because your medications or supplements have rid you of your food obsessions and cravings. At last, you're free to take real control over your life and make choices that are about your health, *not* your weight.

113

12

Exercise to
Feel Great

Exercise won't make you thin. It simply takes too much physical movement to burn off more excess calories than you consume. So why bother exercising at all?

The human body is built to move. It needs to work and play. It has muscles that push, muscles that pull, and a wonderful system for storing fuel for them to burn. When muscles are stressed by pushing or pulling them harder or for a longer time than they're used to, the body builds even more muscle to compensate. That gives you a lean, muscular, athletic body—something that losing weight by dieting alone can't give you.

Exercise has other great benefits, such as improving your self-image, self-confidence, and general sense of well-being. Strenuous activity can make you feel relaxed and good about yourself; it can give you a feeling of accomplishment, of having done a difficult task well. This effect is so strong that in study after study it has actually relieved symptoms of depression in people who are overweight.

Where your general health is concerned, exercise is the closest thing we know to a magic elixir. Statistics show significant increases in longevity among people who are even moderately fit. One Swedish study, for example, showed that female subjects who were most active between the ages of 50 and 74 were 33 percent less likely to die from heart disease. Other studies have shown that exercise reduces the incidence of premature death from other causes as well, such as colon cancer and breast cancer. Research has also demonstrated that the obese and the elderly benefit greatly from exercise.

Of course, before starting any exercise program, be sure to get your doctor's okay.

A QUESTION OF MOTIVATION

An obvious question arises: If exercise is so wonderful, why don't we love to do it? Why don't we wake up in the morning eager to leap onto the stationary bike or to grab hold of a mean-looking set of dumbbells? Three words come to mind: sweaty, painful, boring.

Not everyone feels this way. Many athletes actually do look forward to exercise. So do ordinary folks who have made it part of their daily routine. Their muscles long to stretch and contract the way colts long to romp on the open range. But people who are out of shape, especially if they are also overweight, become disproportionately overstressed with even a small amount of movement. Their muscles are more like old nags than young colts, and chronic dieting has exhausted their systems.

To make matters worse, they feel self-conscious and humiliated wearing workout clothes, such as shorts or tights, most of which are clearly designed to complement lean bodies.

All in all, the pain seems much greater than the gain.

Okay, so, you know it's good for you, but in your heart of hearts, you really, really, *really* don't want to exercise. You know that if you start a program today, in three months you'll get up one morning and say to yourself, "I just can't do it this morning. I'm too tired. I'm too busy. I'm too whatever." You skip that day, and it feels good, so you skip another, and another.

Exercise for Seniors

Aging causes muscles to waste away. Elderly people can find themselves unable to do simple tasks, such as sitting up on their own or walking across a room. The only therapy that works for people in this condition is muscle building, so I took a group of ten people from the nursing home, with an average age of 85, and conducted a weight-lifting class twice a week with them. We used dumbbells ranging from 3 to 5 pounds.

Within a few months, all ten people were all feeling an overall sense of greater strength and improved well-being. One woman gave up her cane as her upper body strength increased. Another was able, for the first time in years, to make her way from her bed to a chair without the aid of a nurse.

Pretty soon you're off your program. You were doing it because everyone told you how good it was for you and how it would keep you younger and stronger.

You had been telling yourself how wonderful it felt to be in better shape. You were telling the truth—to a point. It did feel wonderful, but only after you had gotten the daily routine over with. Before and during, it felt lousy.

So, you really don't want to exercise. Okay, don't—at least for now.

No, I'm not kidding—but I'm not letting you off the hook either.

TAKE SMALL STEPS

As of today, let daily exercise become one of your long-term goals. See it as the finish line. For the moment, you are at the starting gate. Your first step will be to become less sedentary. There is only one unchangeable rule you must remember: For exercise to work, you must always push yourself to do just a little more physical activity than you're used to.

This doesn't mean giving up your desk job or forsaking your life as a homemaker for a career in day labor. It does mean looking for small ways in which you can expend a little more energy. They're easy to find.

Ask yourself some simple questions. Are there places I drive to that I could walk to? When I do drive, could I park a little farther from my destination to give myself the opportunity of walking? When I do walk, could I walk just a little faster? Are there times when I could climb steps rather than ride an escalator or elevator? Could I sometimes wash the dishes by hand rather than use the dishwasher? Can I use a push lawnmower rather than a self-propelled one? If I'm whipping eggs or mixing batter, could I do it by hand rather than using a blender or electric beaters?

Every activity you can think of will use calories, even if only a few, and with time, those calories can add up to substantial amounts.

WHEN YOUR ENGINE STARTS TO HUM

If you have been extremely sedentary, you'll find as you begin to move more that you'll *want* to move more, especially if you have lost 10 or 15 pounds through your Hunger Switch profile program. It feels good to use your muscles, and you'll find yourself growing impatient with sitting around and doing nothing. At this point, you may decide you want to begin a regular exercise program.

All kinds of questions will come up. What is the best program for me? Should I be jogging, lifting weights, doing aerobics, taking up tennis? How often do I need to exercise and for how long? Should I go out and buy expensive equipment? How about special clothing, like sweat pants and running shoes?

My best advice is to calm down. Take it slow. Low-intensity exercise is a perfectly good way to begin, and you're not ready for more yet. Begin with a 15-minute slow walk twice a week. As you feel more and more capable, you can gradually build up to longer treks.

If you're more comfortable indoors than out, or if the weather is a problem, try using a treadmill. Some studies have shown that it is the best indoor aerobic exercise you can do.

Take your walks just after a meal. The body will burn 15 percent more calories if you exercise right after you've eaten. If you exercise just before a meal, on the other hand, you'll dull your appetite a bit, but an hour later you'll rebound and become ravenous. It's not a good idea.

As you continue to become more fit, you may decide to go on to more strenuous exercising. If you do, bear a few facts in mind as you decide which type of program to undertake.

First, aerobic activities such as jogging or playing tennis will not increase your metabolism. If your metabolic rate is slow, it will speed up only during the time that you're exercising. If you want to burn calories and improve the health of your heart, aerobic exercise is great, but don't expect it to deliver more than it can.

Second, resistance exercise, such as weight lifting, will increase your metabolic rate by building more muscle, but it may not burn calories so efficiently while you're doing it. Weight lifting builds muscle. Muscle demands fuel and burns it quickly. Therefore, the metabolic rate goes up. If you add muscle, your body will burn fat at a greater rate every moment of every day.

REVERSING THE DIET EFFECT

If you're young, you may argue that none of this has anything to do with you. An increased metabolic rate would be nice to have, but you're still strong and healthy. Maybe, maybe not.

If you're like most overweight people, you've been on many diets, most of which severely restricted the amount of food you could eat. You lost weight, but what you may not have realized is that much of that weight loss was due to your body cannibalizing your own muscle tissue! The only way around this process is to build new muscle as the old muscle is used up.

The Big Picture

For convenience, here's a summary of the points you should remember about exercise:

- Exercise is better at helping you keep weight off than at making you lose it.

- A little activity is better than nothing. Start slowly, and build up gradually.

- Being overweight and fit is far better than being overweight and out of shape.

- Resistance training with weights will build muscle and help you to keep a strong, fit body, even while you're dieting.

- A combination of aerobics and weight training is ideal.

- A half-hour session, twice per week, of walking, biking, using a treadmill, or jumping rope is the goal you're shooting for.

- A half-hour session of weight training, twice per week, starting out with light weights and attacking only one muscle group at a time, is all you're need of this type of exercise.

- Frequently vary the kinds of exercise you do.

- Don't cut back your calories. Have faith in your medications or natural-supplement program to keep your food intake under control.

A study from the University of Massachusetts demonstrates the point. The subjects were divided into four groups. Here are the results:

- The group that dieted alone lost an average of 9 pounds, but 11 percent of that weight was in the form of muscle.
- The group that dieted and did aerobic exercise lost an average of 10 pounds, but 99 percent of it was fat loss.
- The group that dieted and did strength training lost an average of 9 pounds, but all of the loss was from fat, and some muscle was gained in the process.
- The group that dieted and did both aerobic exercise and resistance training lost an average of 13 pounds, all of it in the form of fat, and gained 4 percent more muscle.

The result is clear: A combination of aerobic exercise and resistance training gives the best benefits. Walking and working out with very light weights is ideal.

Try to work up to two 30-minute aerobic sessions and two 30-minute resistance-training sessions per week. If you're using weights, start with very light weights and exercise one muscle group per week (arms, chest, shoulders, back, etc.).

It's important to make frequent changes in your exercise program. For example, walk for a couple of weeks, then switch to a bike for a couple, then to a treadmill, then to a jump rope. This will keep your body from getting so used to any particular movement that it starts to get easy. You can also vary the intensity of your workout. Some days, walk a little longer or a little faster, or alternate from a quick to slow pace as you go. Constantly changing your workout will put your body into a state of "metabolic panic," which will make it into a much more efficient fat burner.

WATCH WHAT YOU EAT

I would add one note of caution: Don't cut back your calories. Take your medication and eat when you're hungry. You need fuel when you exercise. If you don't have fuel, you'll quickly become fatigued and discouraged. Eat plenty of carbohydrates (vegetables, fruits, and grains) and protein, and keep your fat intake low.

Don't be surprised if you find your weight going up a little. Muscle weighs more than fat, so trust your mirror more than your scale. If you really need numbers to make you feel good, ask your doctor to measure your fat-to-muscle ratio, or to recommend a place where you can have it done. This is sometimes done in a water tank, but usually it's just a matter of measuring your fat folds with a pair of calipers.

13

Our Kids and
Our Parents

Most of us would make any sacrifice to keep our children safe
and healthy. We teach them not to talk to strangers, to look
both ways before crossing the street, and to wash their hands
before eating. We take them to the doctor for immunizations,
earaches, and strep throat.

When they're a little older, we anguish over the dangers
of drugs, sex, and violence. We're on constant lookout for
anything that might threaten their young lives, and we would
lay down our own to protect them.

Why, then, do we ignore a serious and potentially cat-
astrophic problem that affects the lives of a quarter of our
kids?

What am I talking about? A recent edition of the *Archives
of Pediatric and Adolescent Medicine* (March 15, 2001) reported

that we now have twice as many obese children as we did in the previous generation. One child out of every four is dangerously overweight.

Many of these kids will go on to become obese adults. If a child is seriously overweight when 10–13 years old, he or she is six to seven times more likely than other children to have the same problem for the rest of his or her life.

Even those who manage to lose their excess fat by the time they reach maturity aren't out of the woods. Obese children will suffer a greater risk of illness and premature death over the next 50 years of their lives, no matter how thin they become as adults.

No one is sure why obese children tend to become obese adults, or if they don't, why they suffer greater risks to their health. We have, however, identified some factors that increase their risk of obesity and some that do not.

BIRTH WEIGHT

Many things affect how much a child will weigh at birth: Did the baby come before or after the due date? A child gains an ounce per day in the womb during the last month of pregnancy. How big was his or her mother? Genetics plays a significant role. Did the mother smoke during pregnancy? Smoking seems to cause lower birth weight.

One factor that has only a minor role to play is the amount of food a mother eats during pregnancy. Her body will keep the extra calories for itself rather than passing them onto her child.

So long as a baby falls within an average, healthy range of 5.5–9 pounds, birth weight is considered normal.

Even at higher weights, concern is more over complications during delivery than for any health problem the baby may be carrying. There is also no correlation whatsoever between what a person weighs on the first day of his or her life and what he or she will weigh on the 21st anniversary of that day.

In fact, that correlation doesn't occur until adolescence. It is the 10- to 13-year-old for whom we are most concerned.

FAT CELLS

The total number of fat cells a person develops from age 10 to 13 may have something to do with the problem, but even this is controversial. Most people will end up with 120 to 160 billion fat cells in their bodies by the time they reach adulthood. Usually, that number is set during or just after adolescence. It would seem logical to conclude that the more fat cells you have, the fatter you will likely be.

Not the case. Fat cells are like deflated balloons. They take up very little space. Fill them with fat, however, and they'll blow up very big. So it's the *size* of the fat cells, *not* their number, which is significant. That means you can have relatively few fat cells and still be obese. On the other hand, you can have many, many fat cells and never put on a pound of excess weight in your life.

WHAT TO DO

Modifying some of these risk factors may help children to maintain a healthy weight throughout their lives. Ignoring them, on the other hand, may lead to all sorts of health problems.

Seriously overweight children enter puberty sooner, have a shorter period of bone growth, and are at greater risk for high blood pressure, elevated cholesterol levels, orthopedic problems, and menstrual problems. Just as important, their self-image can become seriously distorted, leading to depression and worse.

This is especially true among teenage girls. Eight out of ten, when polled, say they need to lose weight and would like to talk to a doctor about diet and exercise. Unfortunately, most are too intimidated to do so.

Fat Television

Dr. William Dietz of the Harvard School of Public Health has discovered an interesting risk factor for children being overweight. There is a direct correlation between the number of hours a child sits and watches television and the degree to which he or she is obese.

Some of the reasons for this are obvious. Watching television is sedentary. People tend to consume more junk food as they watch. Advertisements for food may cause people to head for the refrigerator more often. But Dr. Dietz has offered another, more subtle, reason: Watching television leads the viewer into a trance-like state that may have the effect of slowing down the metabolism! The explanation that makes more sense to me is that this trance is like the hypnotic state, which raises serotonin levels without raising norepinephrine—a surefire way to gain weight.

WHAT CAN WE DO?

I have found over the past several years that weight loss in adolescents can be as difficult to achieve as it is in adults. Again, the problem is mostly due to a genetic predisposition that leads to imbalances in brain chemistry. Diets and activity won't bring about permanent weight loss.

I must admit that this is a very tough problem. Some physicians prescribe low doses of phentermine with very good results and few side effects. I have used this approach with kids 16 years and older, but I haven't tried it with patients younger than this. I don't have enough scientific data or experience to recommend the Hunger Switch approach for younger teenagers; however, I believe it will eventually prove their most effective—and perhaps only—method of achieving long-term weight loss.

Until more studies have been done, your only option is to try traditional methods of weight control. If you can achieve any degree of success, you'll at least have done something to help your child. Here some approaches you can try.

- **Reduce fat.** Cut down on the fatty foods your child eats, especially fast foods. This doesn't mean eliminating red meat and French fries from the diet altogether. Kids won't tolerate that. As in all things, moderation is the key.

- **Cut sweets.** You can reduce your child's snacking and desserts, but again, don't be too rigid or strict. Try substituting high-fat desserts with their low-fat counterparts, but remember that overindulging in anything that contains a lot of sugar, even low-fat foods, will put on weight.

- **Push protein.** Feed your child more lean protein, fruit, whole grains, vegetables, and low-fat dairy products. It's not enough to get rid of the bad things in your child's diet. You have to replace them with good things.

- **Encourage exercise.** Get your child to be more active on a day-to-day basis. Encourage your child to climb stairs, do yard work, walk a little more, and anything else you can think of to keep him or her moving. Start your child in an exercise program. Swimming, biking, running, and jumping rope are all good choices, but whatever the activity, it should be done four times a week in 20-minute sessions. Kids find this kind of routine easier to follow when the entire family is involved, so parents and siblings will have a good opportunity to get in shape as well!

OLDER FOLKS

Children, of course, are not the only people we love who come under our care. So do our aging parents and grandparents.

For too long a time, the attitude among physicians was that the elderly didn't need aggressive treatment for health problems. They weren't going to live long anyway, so why risk making their lives miserable with side effects from drugs?

To the credit of the medical profession, this attitude has changed, largely in response to research. Your family doctor now realizes that elderly patients benefit greatly from aggressive treatment of heart disease, diabetes, hypertension, and elevated cholesterol levels. They also get great results with exercise programs, whether for improving aerobic capacity or for increasing muscle strength.

I'm convinced that elderly patients could enjoy healthier, longer lives if we also took an aggressive approach to helping them control their weight.

Of course, our concerns are the same as they are in treating any illness in this age group: drug/supplement interactions, coinciding illnesses, and dosage.

Because older people are more sensitive to medications in general, elderly patients should start their regimen at the lowest possible doses and, if necessary, work gradually upward.

Consistent exercise will also help to vastly improve the quality of life for people in their later years. Building muscle will make them feel stronger, boost their sense of well being, and make them more mobile. They'll also suffer from fewer falls and fractures. I wouldn't be surprised if their improved health allowed them to stop taking many of their other medications, which in turn would mean fewer side effects.

Overall, I look for a picture of much better health among our very young and very old as we bring their weight problems under control, but they are not the only population groups we need to single out for special attention.

14

Special Advice for Men

Men can use all of the information and advice in this book, but they're not likely to. In fact, it's hard to imagine a more uncooperative, unwilling patient than the average American male. Even if he's obviously ill, he'll resist doing anything about it until his symptoms get so bad they interfere with his work. Mention his weight to him and you're lucky if he so much as loosens his belt a notch.

So if you're a woman, just how do you get your husband, father, son, uncle, or brother to pay attention to what's clearly a health risk, as well as an appearance issue?

If a rash, fever, or elevated temperature won't drive a man to change his ways, how on Earth do you get him to do so just because his pants don't fit like they used to? This chapter is designed to help you do exactly that.

MOVING THE MOUNTAIN

If he's like most men, it is only when his weight begins to interfere with his day-to-day life by making him fatigued, sluggish, and short of breath after minimal exertion that he will actually consider seeing a professional. Even then, he may remain stubborn. It may take the onset of diabetes, arthritis, or some other weight-related illness to move him.

This, of course, is not an acceptable situation. Here's what to try.

Tell Him What You See

Make him aware that you notice he's overweight. He may not be paying attention to his shape, but he will if he knows you are. At the same time, let him know that you're not criticizing him, but rather that you're concerned about his health. Point out that his apple-shaped physique (big belly, small hips), which is typical of the overweight male, has proven in study after study to pose far more of a health risk than does the pear-shaped physique (smaller belly, larger hips and buttocks) of the overweight female.

Share Your Successes

If you've lost weight yourself recently, or have done something else to significantly improve your appearance, let him know how good it makes you feel to look younger, healthier, and more attractive. Tell him you want the same things for him. He'll want to look better for you at first, but as he begins to have some success with his weight-loss program, he'll also want to look better for himself.

List the Professional Advantages

Gently point out that losing weight may help him in his job, especially if his work requires contact with clients or the general public. He may have already thought about this on his own. As a man grows older, he begins to realize that his younger counterparts have their eyes on his job or sometimes his clients. In a case such as this, a better appearance can mean the difference between success or failure in his career.

Tell Him the Benefits

Point out that he'll feel better in general if he sheds his excess weight and gets into better shape. No one likes becoming short of breath and exhausted just from moving about the house or going up a flight of stairs. There's hardly a man alive who wouldn't prefer to have the energy, strength, and vigor to work all day, come home and play with his kids, go out for the evening to have a good time with the woman he loves, then come home with energy to spare for some bedroom romance.

THE UPSIDES AND DOWNSIDES OF BEING A MALE

Men suffer a health disadvantage because of the way in which fat tends to collect around their abdomens rather than their hips and buttocks. On the other hand, their metabolism gives them a big advantage once they decide to get rid of that fat.

Because of his higher testosterone level, the average male will have significantly greater muscle mass than the average female. This greater muscle mass, in turn, allows him to lift heavier weights and work against greater resistance, which creates even more muscle mass. Since muscle cells are efficient fat burners 24 hours per day, all of this muscle helps him to lose weight more quickly than his female counterpart.

If men have all these advantages when it comes to losing weight, why should they be concerned about medications or supplements?

There is one aspect of dieting at which men do not do well: portion control. What comes to mind when you think of a "man-size" meal? Enough food to feed a horse. The healthiest, leanest food in the world will put fat on you if you eat too much of it.

Thus, appetite control is a major issue for men. The best way to control appetite, as we've seen, is to use the right tools to move the internal thermostat and turn off the hunger switch.

BODY-BUILDING SUPPLEMENTS

Men like to putter, fix, and improve. Very often, as soon as a man begins to experience some success with a project, he immediately starts looking for ways to get even better results. This is usually the point at which he asks me about supplements that can help him boost his energy and muscle mass. These are the ones I'm usually asked about.

DHEA

If he's done any research on his own, the first supplement he will ask about is DHEA (dehydroepiandosterone), a steroid hormone that's supposed to do everything from curing cancer to reversing the aging process.

What's This I Hear About GHB?

Whatever you've heard, GHB is nasty stuff. In addition to its well-known use as a "date-rape" drug because it produces an alcohol-like inebriation, men have been using it as a body-building supplement. Bad move. It turns out that the stuff is highly addictive and leads to very serious withdrawal symptoms—serious enough to land many men in the hospital. The symptoms—which include anxiety, insomnia, tremor, hallucinations, psychotic behavior requiring sedation and restraints, delirium, and loss of control of the autonomic nervous system—can last up to two weeks. In at least one case, withdrawal has led to death. The same dangers hold true for GHB's chemical relatives, butyrolactone and butanediol.

How many of these claims are true has yet to be seen. Not enough research has been done. We do know, however, that DHEA reduces body fat and raises metabolism, even when taken in doses as low as 10–25 mg per day. If supplements prove safe for human use, they could be a valuable addition to a weight-loss program . . . but that's a big "if."

DHEA occurs naturally in the body, but in tiny amounts. No one knows what adding more of the chemical to the metabolic mix will do in the long term. My advice for now is to wait and see what the research eventually shows. If a man decides to use DHEA in spite of the risks, he should at least have his blood levels checked first, and talk over his decision with his doctor.

Testosterone

Supplementing with the male hormone testosterone also shows promise as an aid to men who are trying to lose weight and build healthier bodies. Testosterone will give you more muscle and greater strength, increase your sex drive, and improve your memory. On the other hand, it can lead to aggressive behavior and prostate problems, so most doctors will insist on taking a blood level first, then supplement with doses based on the results.

We're still in the early stages of learning how to use testosterone effectively, but it shows real promise, especially for men over 60 years of age.

HGH

The most promising of any of these substances is HGH, or human growth hormone. It not only lowers body fat and increases muscle mass, but it also increases blood levels of the so-called "good" HDL cholesterol (high-density lipoprotein) and improves bone density. While at higher doses it can lead to high blood pressure and diabetes, at appropriate doses of about 1.5 mg per day it actually lowers blood pressure and strengthens the heart. I have very high hope for HGH as a weapon in the fight against body fat.

If a man has a well-rounded diet that includes plenty of different fruits and vegetables, it probably isn't necessary for him to take a daily multivitamin supplement. However, I would suggest taking a good assortment of antioxidants. This is good advice for women, as well.

Antioxidants are substances that neutralize "free radicals," particles that roam around the body doing all sorts of damage at the molecular level and are responsible, at least in part, for aging and many diseases.

It's especially important to take antioxidants if you exercise vigorously. Tissue breakdown that occurs during exercise raises the level of free radicals in the body, so it's important to offset this effect with supplements.

Here's what I recommend:

- Vitamin E as alpha tocopherol: 400 IU per day
- Selenium: 200 mcg per day
- Pycnogenol: 30 mg per day
- Folic acid: 400 mcg per day
- Zinc: 60 mg per day.

It's better not to buy a general antioxidant that contains all of these ingredients, as it's nearly impossible to get the recommended doses of each substance into one or two pills. Buy them separately, but remember that more expensive does not necessarily mean higher quality. Shop for price and quality. Look for brands that don't contain added sugar, yeast, or coloring. Don't forget to look over mail order catalogs and Web sites, which are excellent ways to buy supplements at a reasonable cost.

15

Common Questions with Uncommon Answers

Among the many questions I've had from patients over the years are a few that come up over and over again. Some of them have undoubtedly occurred to you. I hope the following discussions will be helpful.

Q. Am I overweight because of poor eating behavior or heredity?

A. Both. Several studies have demonstrated conclusively that genetics exerts a strong influence over the tendency to gain weight (see Chapter 3). On the other hand, many other studies have shown that the amount of fat you eat also plays a role in determining how fat you become. This may seem contradictory, but it isn't. Heredity studies tell us that a person's genetic background will determine how likely it is that he or she will become obese, as compared with the rest of the population. Fat intake, however, helps to determine how fat any individual actually becomes. Heredity gives the odds; environment determines the real life outcome. It's like a horse race: Theoretically, the thoroughbred with the strongest lineage should win every race, but anything from track conditions to the temperament of the jockey can change the outcome.

Q. If being overweight is a result of both heredity and environment, what does an imbalance in my brain chemistry have to do with it?

A. An imbalance of certain biochemicals in the brains of overweight people is an inherited condition and is largely responsible for the food obsessions and cravings that drive you to eat too much. It's virtually impossible to control these cravings for any length of time by willpower alone. That's where the use of medications come in. The pills restore a proper chemical balance to the brain, which in turn, relieves you of cravings and allows you to comfortably reduce the amount of food you eat, especially fat.

Q. If genetics causes me to be fat, why was I a thin child and teenager?

A. Most often, genes don't express themselves until later in life. People with highly hereditary diseases, such as diabetes, high blood pressure, and even cancer, usually develop them as adults when a stressful life event stimulates a genetic dysfunction. The event may be an emotional stressor, pregnancy, change in career or marriage, death of a loved one, or even a new medication. These things can trigger the genetic process that leads to imbalance in your brain chemistry, which moves up the brain thermostat and flips on the hunger switch causing uncontrolled weight gain.

Q. What can I do when my weight loss just stops?

A. This can be a difficult problem since it is hard to know if the brain has reached a new set point or a temporary plateau. I always change medication at this point and sometimes the approach is successful. But if you've arrived at a new set point, your weight will probably not drop further, because you've reached your ideal weight—no matter what the insurance charts say. Your brain determines your particular ideal body weight. It doesn't care what the average weight is for your height; it will take you where it wants you to go and even medications will not push it further.

Q. Do I have to stay on pills forever?

A. Most people, but not all, need some kind of maintenance dose. A few are able maintain weight loss through diet and exercise. More often than not, however, once the pills stop, the brain thermostat starts to move upward and the lost pounds return. Fortunately, taking medications just three times a week in accordance with a doctor's recommendations can adequately maintain weight loss, especially when combined with very moderate lifestyle changes.

Q. Can you be too thin?

A. Certainly anorexia is too thin and very dangerous. Not eating at all is obviously unhealthy and can lead to serious illness and sudden death. But the fact is that very lean men and women statistically live the longest. A study of 62,000 men and 260,000 women showed that the very thin, with BMIs of only 19 to 22, had the lowest risk of premature death from any cause. This is a very lean weight, but not model thin. Monkeys that are fed a low-calorie diet and are leaner than others often live twice as long as their heavier counterparts. Thin is healthy—but not to the point of starvation.

Q. How much of a problem does obesity really create?

A. Every year, obesity is responsible for over $70 billion in health-care costs and 300,000 deaths in the United States alone. It contributes to heart disease, high blood pressure, stroke, breast and colon cancers, some forms of diabetes, gallbladder disease, and lung disease. Only smoking is more dangerous.

144

Q. What do I do if phentermine or ephedra "wire me"?

A. Ask your doctor for a very low dose of the beta blocker Pindolol®. Two to five milligrams does a great job in stopping the stimulant effects of these agents, even insomnia, without side effects. It's also very inexpensive, but you'll need a prescription to buy it. Over-the-counter kavakava can be helpful but requires patience since it doesn't work immediately. Be careful to get a product that is a 200-mg dose with 30-percent karalactones. Dose is one to three daily.

Q. Is childhood overeating a serious risk later in life?

A. Unfortunately, it can be a serious risk. If a child consumes 240 excess calories daily, his or her cancer risk as an adult increases 15 to 20 percent, and the risk rises even higher as the number of daily calories goes up. Overeating can be very difficult to control, since brain chemistry imbalances are driving up the child's appetite and cravings. Once again, this is not a matter of willpower, but we don't want to put children on medications or supplements either. How to deal with this problem in children is obviously highly controversial.

Q. What are realistic weight-loss expectations?

A. Bariatricians consider a weight loss of 10 percent of body weight a success—especially if it can be maintained. This translates into a loss of 25 pounds for a

250-pound woman. Most people would find this result disappointing. In fact, studies show that the average 250-pound woman would only be happy with a 55- to 77-pound weight loss. While this is very understandable, it's not particularly realistic in all cases.

Q. Can stress cause weight gain?

A. Absolutely. Even without changing your eating behavior, stress will cause weight gain. It is so powerful that even with medications, weight will go up. This is due to the tremendous release of stress hormones, in particular one called cortisol . Interestingly, this kind or stress response is most common in people who are already overweight. Thin people will often stop eating and lose weight under stress. Again, this represents a difference in brain chemistry and is clearly not a function of willpower or self-control.

Q. Is seasonal depression related to increased food cravings in fall and winter months?

A. You may have seen articles in the popular press about something called "seasonal affective disorder" (SAD), which is a state of depression that begins in autumn, gradually worsens during winter, and disappears with the advent of spring. Research has shown that this depression coincides with a drop in serotonin levels. The theory states that fewer hours of

daylight at this time of year trigger a serotonin-spar-
ing response in the brain. That would certainly
explain why these people show such marked
improvement when they use Prozac®, a drug that
increases serotonin levels. Many also experience an
increase in cravings and food obsessions during the
fall and winter. Although we have traditionally
blamed seasonal weight gain on holiday meals, it may
be that changing balances of brain chemistry increase
food cravings as well as depression.

**Q. Does taking estrogen pills make weight loss more
difficult?**

A. Yes. Estrogen promotes fat storage, which really isn't
surprising when you think about it. The hormones a
woman's body naturally produces are designed to
prepare you for pregnancy and childbirth. This
means storing fat, especially in the hips and thighs.
Unfortunately, your body doesn't know the difference between a supplement and natural estrogen, so
if you're taking this medication, you will probably
have more difficulty in losing weight.

**Q. Why do my food cravings get so intense right before
menstruation?**

A. Once again, serotonin is the answer. Levels drop in
the premenstrual phase of your cycle. Because serotonin is the chemical that keeps you calm, not having
enough of it causes you to get irritable and anxious—
and to crave sweets and starches.

Q. What about the use of fluid pills or diuretics for weight control?

A. There are absolutely no indications for the use of diuretics in a weight-loss program, and they can dangerously lower your blood pressure and potassium levels. Remember, losing fluid is not the same as losing fat. If you sweat out 8 ounces of perspiration when you exercise, you'll gain it back with your next glass of water. If you're trying to lose weight, diuretics are not an option. (Of course, doctors prescribe diuretics for other health conditions, and you should not discontinue prescription diuretics unless you talk to your physician.)

Q. Do you use any behavior-modification techniques?

A. Behavior modification for obesity can be broken down into three steps. First, you must identify those factors that lead to overeating, such as particularly tempting foods, emotional stress, social situations, and so on. Next, put obstacles and distractions on the road between temptation and giving in. For example, if you find yourself mesmerized by the dessert buffet at a wedding reception, you might step outside for a walk, drink a very large glass of water, or find a partner and dance that polka the band is playing. Finally, you reward yourself for a job well done and give yourself a little pat on the back whenever you resist a particularly strong temptation.

Behavior modification is great as part of an overall program. By itself, however, it yields disappointing results because it treats symptoms rather than the underlying illness. It does not make food obsessions and cravings go away, and people who suffer under the assault of these impulses twenty-four hours a day are likely to give in sooner or later. That means the weight comes back. In my opinion, the problem of brain-serotonin levels must be addressed.

Q. Do weight-loss medications and supplements work for everyone?

A. In my experience, low doses of weight-loss medications are effective in about 95 percent of patients. "Effective" means that the average patient will lose 10 percent of his or her starting body weight in three to six months. In my experience, the patient who does not lose weight on the Hunger Switch program is very rare indeed.

Q. How do I set my goal weight?

A. To be frank, I don't think setting a goal weight is a good idea. It's too easy to set yourself up for failure with unrealistic expectations. Instead, every pound lost should be cause for celebration. Losing 20 pounds will give you significant health benefits and a much-improved image of yourself. If you're 100–150 pounds overweight, don't even worry about your ideal body weight. Getting there may not be reasonable and probably isn't necessary. If you lose 10 percent of your body weight and keep it off in the long term, you have, in my opinion, accomplished something great.

Having said all this, I realize that many people will insist upon having a way to know when they've lost enough weight. Okay, then, here it is: Listen to your own body. After you have been taking medications for awhile—no one can predict for how long— you will reach a plateau in your weight loss. Nothing you do—not limiting calories, stopping and restarting your medications, or raising their dosages—will budge the scale. Your body will be telling you that it's at the weight it prefers. Only very extreme, almost obsessive exercising will make any more weight come off. If there is any such thing as a goal or ideal or baseline weight, this is the way in which you will know you have reached it.

Q. Can being overweight lead to arthritis and other painful problems?

A. Unfortunately, yes. We have long suspected that the extra stress and strain inflicted on the joints of overweight people might cause inflammation or arthritis. Recently, a study done by Dr. Allan Gelber, a rheumatologist at Johns Hopkins, confirmed our suspicions. Men who are even moderately overweight are at significantly greater risk for arthritis of the hips and knees. Gelber's study focused on osteoarthritis, which is a painful joint condition that results from the loss of cartilage, a tissue that acts as a shock absorber for the bones. When cartilage wears thin, the joints become warm, swollen, stiff, and painful. The condition afflicts about a third of all people over the age of 65, but appears in overweight people far sooner—sometimes as early as 20 years of age.

Q. Should I totally avoid fatty foods?

A. No. In fact, it's not a good idea. You need small amounts of fatty acids to maintain good health. But even if you could avoid them, would you want to? Do you really want to give up all of your favorite foods? You need to indulge yourself now and then, to give yourself some pleasure. One of the reasons these medications and natural supplements work so well is that they allow you to eat "junk" food now and then without worry. The difference will be that you won't feel any need to overeat. You'll find you can enjoy a few potato chips or a single scoop of ice cream and be satisfied.

Q. What medications are weight gainers?

A. Many! The biggest offenders are antihistamines, used for allergies; antiseizure drugs; beta blockers, used for hypertension and migraines; estrogen; and almost all antidepressants, unless they're used with phentermine. Furthermore, weight gain can occur very rapidly from the brain-chemistry changes induced by these medications. This sets off the entire genetic cascade of events leading to significant weight gain. Unfortunately, drug-induced weight gain is extremely difficult to take off without the help of medications. This particular problem is very frustrating, since the medication is often vital for the patient's overall health. I have found that weight-loss medications are the only answer to this dilemma. In any case, you should never discontinue the use of the weight-gain drugs I have mentioned unless you consult your doctor.

Q. This is confusing because I've heard that Prozac® will make you lose weight. Is this true?

A. Prozac® can have that effect for the initial two or three months. Weight gain almost always occurs after that period. But some of the other SSRIs, such as Paxil®, are even worse.

Q. What about blood-pressure medications and weight gain?

A. Some notorious weight gainers are the diuretics like hydrochlorothiazide, the calcium channel blocker verapamil, and the beta blockers like propanolol and atanolol. Good alternatives are the ace-inhibitors (of which there are many), which are relatively side-effect free, easy to use, and inexpensive. The beta blocker Pindolol® is also a very good choice. But of course you need to talk to your doctor while considering these alternatives.

Q. What can I take for allergies?

A. Beware of all antihistamines—even the newer ones. They're weight gainers. If you're using over-the-counter anti-histamines to treat allergy symptoms, try a local steroid nasal spray. Use Sudafed™ for congestion and Tylenol™ for discomfort. Ask your doctor about the various eyedrops available for itchy eyes. Daily antihistamines are particularly troublesome.

Q. Can I use any antidepressants and not gain weight?

A. Wellbutrin® is probably the safest, so far as gaining weight is concerned, but it isn't for everyone. People with seizures can't use it, and it sometimes "wires" people too much. Also, it doesn't raise serotonin levels, so it's not always an ideal antidepressant. Again, if you have a weight problem and your doctor has recommended that you use a serotonin antidepressant, phentermine should be used along with it. Pindolol® at 4 mg per day is also a serotonin agent, which helps with depression and stops the anxiety that occasionally accompanies phentermine. It's a beta blocker and is good for blood-pressure control, as well as panic that accompanies public speaking.

Author's Note

Ephedra *(ma huang)* is perhaps one of the most controversial weight loss products in recent history. I'm often asked about its safety, as the media seems to release a new story about the dangers of the substance almost daily. To shed some light on the issue, I've asked for an opinion from James R. Prochnow, J.D., an attorney who has defended ephedra products in many major cases brought by the Food and Drug Administration. I've included Jim's research and opinion not as a blanket recommendation of ephedra for everyone, and not to offer medical or legal advice to anyone, but to inform the reader regarding the issues surrounding this controversial weight-loss product so that readers can draw their own conclusions regarding the use of ephedra. As with any weight-loss medication, supplement, or program, ephedra products should be used in any particular case only after consultation with a qualified health care professional. If anyone knows where ephedra stands, both with regard to safety and its legal use, Jim does. As he concludes, the study of adverse reactions by the FDA (by its own admission) is neither complete nor thorough enough to warrant withdrawal of this product from the market. As I've noted previously, none of my patients have noted any ill effects when using the small amounts of ephedra I prescribe.

Afterword

How Safe Is Ma Huang?

Regulation of Ephedra in the U.S.

by James R. Prochnow, J.D.

Ma huang, commonly referred to as ephedra, has been included as a botanical ingredient in dietary supplements since, at least, the late 1970s. In the United States, as contrasted with ephedra's traditional use in China for medicinal purposes, ephedra supplements have been promoted by companies and used by consumers as a means to achieve weight maintenance or loss and to feel energized. Ephedra is not commonly included as an ingredient in foods that are not dietary supplements, called common or conventional foods, because it is not an approved food additive and, at least to date, does not have formal GRAS (Generally Recognized as Safe) status. Neither of those food classifications is applicable to dietary supplements. Because of its use as a food or food ingredient before October 15, 1994, ephedra is not classified as a new dietary ingredient, which would require pre-market notice to the Food and Drug Administration (FDA), including reasonable evidence of safety.

The regulation of dietary supplements that contain ephedra is the responsibility of the FDA and comparable state food and drug agencies. Until recently, however, the FDA has shouldered virtually the entire regulatory burden. States have taken a much more active role in the 1995–2000 period, due to the FDA's allocation of scarce resources to nonfood issues, the abundance of news stories about rumors of serious injuries and deaths from ephedra dietary supplements, and the ability of states to expand their regulatory operations thanks to excess revenue.

The FDA, on June 4, 1997, published a Proposed Rule (a proposed federal regulation) that would probably reduce sales of ephedra products. The substance of and impetus for the FDA's decision to issue such a regulation have been the target of several congressional hearings, extensive mass-media coverage, and intensive scientific and industry lobbying. The Proposed Rule was substantially withdrawn by the FDA on April 3, 2000; as of May 1, 2001, the FDA had not promulgated any legally binding federal regulation that directly affects ephedra products.

GENERAL INFORMATION ABOUT THE USE OF EPHEDRA IN DIETARY SUPPLEMENTS

Dietary supplements that contain ephedra are often referred to as ephedra products or ephedra dietary supplements or as ephedrine alkaloid-containing supplements because the most dominant ingredient in ephedra is ephedrine. In the United

States, the dietary ingredient that delivers ephedrine to the body consists, most often, of a 6-percent or 8-percent powder extract of the ephedra herb.

Occasionally, ephedrine hydrochloride (EHCL), whether ultimately derived from a natural source or totally made from chemicals in a manufacturing facility, is the source of the ephedrine. The Dietary Supplement Health and Education Act of 1994 (DSHEA) does not prohibit the use of EHCL, regardless of its "natural" or artificial source, in dietary supplements, but several states' laws or regulations do. The typical ephedra-containing product contains about 12 milligrams (mg) of ephedrine alkaloids per unit, whether that unit is in the form of a liquid, tablet, capsule or caplet, and commonly contains 24 mg per serving.

Ephedra is often combined with caffeine, from an herb such as kola nut or guarana, in a typical ephedra product. Either alone or when combined with a caffeine-containing herb or plant, ephedra, due to its ephedrine content, stimulates the sympathetic nerve system and evokes a response in the consumer that he or she can readily feel.

HISTORY OF TRADITIONAL USE IN CHINA AND OTHER COUNTRIES

Dr. Dennis Jones, a distinguished scientist in the dietary supplement industry, submitted extensive historical data on the historical use of ephedra in an October 9, 1995 submission to the FDA Committee on Food Products. He said:

> The oldest current record of man's interest in Ephedra dates back approximately 20,000 years, to the burial of a Neanderthal individual in what is now Iraq (Lietava,

159

1992), who was buried with a number of plants, including Ephedra altissima.

Under the name Ma huang, Ephedra has traditionally been used in China as an invigorating tea or infusion with beneficial effects on respiration for more than 5000 years (Stuart, 1979), and the earliest written reference to its use and properties is attributed by some experts to the Emperor, Shen Nung (circa 3100 B.C.) in what may have been the first ever Pharmacopoeia, the *Ben Cao Chien* (others claim that the Shen Nung Ben Cao Chien did not appear until about 100 B.C.). This work was substantially revised and enlarged by Li Shih-Chen (1596).

The Indo-Aryans knew Ephedra as an edible plant that gave strength and happiness, and combated exhaustion (Mahdihassan, 1981). Though Indo-Aryans traditionally believed that substances conferring longevity were mainly inorganic, Ephedra was considered as a food with similar beneficial properties (Mahdihassan, 1984), and there is strong evidence that the Rigveda references to *soma* actually describe Ephedra juice (Mahdihassan and Mehdi, 1989). Soma, according to the Rigveda, was the drink of longevity which was even given to newborn infants; this Aryan custom was later to be followed by the Romans, and is still practiced among the Parsee of Bombay and in parts of Iran. Lewis and Elvin-Lewis (1977) also report a long history of use of the dried stems of Ephedra gerardiana in Northern India and Pakistan.

Ephedra was well known to the Romans, and was clearly described by Gaius Plinius Secundus in 77 A.D. (see Rackham et al., 1956–1966) in his *Natural History*, a work that encompassed 37 volumes, of which 12 dealt solely with the healing properties of plants! The herb was apparently not widely used in Europe after the times of the Romans (Moritz, 1953), though sporadic references do occur in medieval European literature; Gerard (1597), for example, refers to Herba Ephedrae (presumed to be Ephedra fragilis) as the "Great shrubbie sea Grape."

In North America, historical use of Ephedra species is well-documented (Kowalchik and Hylton, 1987; Moerman, 1986; Rose, 1972; Saunders, 1920; Tyler, 1982). Traditional users of Ephedra herb recommend dosages that are in excess of those given for ephedrine or pseudoephedrine in pharmaceutical forms, and are also very much higher than those recommended for Dietary Supplements containing Ma huang in the United States. For example, according to Chinese reference works (such as Ou Ming, 1989), Ma huang proper is generally given 3 times daily as a decoction of 3–10 grams of the stems, corresponding to a daily range of 112–180 mg alkaloids at the low end to 375–600 mg alkaloids at the high end, assuming that the Ma huang would contain 1.25%–2% total alkaloids.

The British Herbal Pharmacopoeia (1983) is somewhat more conservative, but still recommends a dose of 1–4 grams 3 times daily (thus 125–500 mg alkaloids per day), for a herb with a minimum alkaloid content of 1.25%.

These relatively high dosages may be explained by the fact that the herb does not behave like pure ephedrine alkaloids; for example, according to the British Herbal Pharmacopoeia (1983), *Ephedra herb does not have the marked pressor effect of ephedrine.* This appears to be due to slower absorption of the alkaloids from the herb than from pharmaceutical formulations (Harada and Nishimura, 1981; Reid, 1986), so there is no sudden rush of ephedrine into the body. The differences between pure ephedrine and Ma huang also show up in formal animal safety studies. Minamatsu et al. (1991) compared pure ephedrine with an extract of Ma huang, and concluded that the extract was less lethal. They also noted that while animals that died after ephedrine administration showed histological changes in some organs, these changes were not found in animals that died after large doses of extract, suggestive of lower classical toxicity.

While most attention has been focused on medicinal use of Ephedra herb, Tanaka (1976) describes Ephedra as a food plant, and Katiyar et al. (1990) report use of parts of the plant as food in some Himalayan tribes. The USDA (1937) classified Ephedra as a highly beneficial forage crop, and allowing meat and milk animals to graze on Ephedra apparently improves meat and milk quality and quantity as well as overall health of the animals (Kovacevic et al., 1974).

Ephedrine has been available in Germany since 1896 and in the U.S. since 1926 (Chen and Schmidt, *Ephedrine and Related Substances*, Baltimore 1930). In 1926, ephedrine was approved for sale in the U.S. by the American Medical Association.

REGULATION OF EPHEDRA BY AND AFTER DSHEA

All dietary supplements are regulated by reference to the Dietary Supplement Health and Education Act of 1994 (DSHEA). Regulations are issued by the FDA to implement that statute and by other provisions of the Federal Food, Drug, and Cosmetic Act. DSHEA, popularly called the "Bill of Rights" for the dietary supplement industry, became effective on October 25, 1994. Among many of its controversial provisions are Section 4, which established safety standards for all dietary supplements, and Section 3, which, for the first time, defined "Dietary Supplement." Prior to then, the phrase "food supplement" was commonly used.

The breadth of that definition has generated considerable debate and has frustrated the policymakers and enforcement arms of the FDA. It is, however, consistent with the legislative objectives of Senator Orrin Hatch (R-Utah), the very visible champion of this industry, and with the extensive Congressional findings which, in Section 2 of that Act, emphasize the need for increased consumer access to information about food supplements and to supplements themselves.

Ironically, 1994 not only marked the beginning of the modern era of dietary supplements and freer access to all supplements, including those that contain ephedra, but the beginning of: (a) a wave of product liability lawsuits against the distributors and manufacturers of ephedra products, and (b) FDA regulatory actions designed to eliminate or significantly restrict their availability to minors and the general population.

From 1995 to date, many states have enacted statutes and issued regulations that, for the most part, restrict the quantity of ephedrine that can be delivered to consumers in a single serving or on a daily basis, limit the promotional claims that can be made about these products, and require that specified warnings be on the label and prohibit the use of EHCL.

Below, you will find references to those who participate at various stages of developing and selling ephedra products. Among them are formulators, raw ingredient suppliers, suppliers of other components (such as labels and containers), manufacturers (who blend, bottle, label, and package ingredients), marketers, distributors and salespersons. Throughout this discussion, the term "distributor" will be used to describe the entity that is primarily responsible for the claims being made about the product and that asserts ownership of the product.

FEDERAL AND STATE STANDARDS OF SAFETY

Almost all product liability claims based on the ingestion of dietary supplements involve ephedra products. Therefore, it is very important for manufacturers, distributors, and suppliers of such products to be aware of the scope of their duty to present only safe products to consumers.

The major federal law that addresses the safety of dietary supplements is Section 4 of DSHEA, now codified at 21 U.S.C. Sec._342 (f) (1). It reads, in pertinent, part:

> A product shall be deemed to be adulterated (i.e., unsafe) if it is a dietary supplement or contains a dietary ingredient that—
>
> (A)   presents a significant or unreasonable risk of illness or injury under—
>
>   (i)   conditions of use recommended or suggested in labeling; or
>
>   (ii)   if no conditions of use are suggested or recommended in the labeling, under ordinary conditions of use;

(B)   is a new dietary ingredient for which there is inadequate information to provide reasonable assurance that such ingredient does not present a significant or unreasonable risk of illness or injury;

(C)   the Secretary declares to pose an imminent hazard to the public health or safety;

(D)   is or contains a dietary ingredient that renders it adulterated under paragraph (a)(1) 21 U.S.C. §342 under the conditions of use recommended or suggested in the labeling of such dietary supplement.

In any proceeding under this subparagraph, the United States shall bear the burden of proof on each element to show that a dietary supplement is adulterated. The court shall decide any issue under this paragraph on a *de novo* basis.

DSHEA compels the FDA to proceed against individual products when it believes a safety issue exists, as contrasted with proceeding against a class of supplements, such as "all ephedra products." An open issue is whether this statute must or should be applied by federal and state courts when the safety of a supplement is in issue.

No court has decided that Sec. 4 of DSHEA supersedes, replaces, or preempts the laws of the 50 states. Therefore, to date, the legal standards used by courts and juries in all or virtually all state and federal civil lawsuits for money damages are standards developed by state legislatures and courts, not by the FDA or the Congress. The standard used in these types of cases varies according to which state's law is being applied by the trial judge and which theories or principles of liability are pursued by legal counsel for a particular consumer.

Nonetheless, there does exist a common, general principle among all of these state standards. That principle, when
applied to a seller of a dietary supplement, is that a seller is
liable to an injured consumer if a finder of fact, such as a jury
or judge, concludes that some condition of the product ren-
dered it unreasonably dangerous. Among other things, failure to give an adequate warning to consumers could render
the product "unreasonably dangerous."

Many facts are relevant to such a determination.
Therefore, it is necessary for any company that distributes
ephedra products to understand, thoroughly, the nature and
characteristics of each dietary ingredient in the product and
the effects on the human body of the product as a whole.

SPECIAL CONSIDERATIONS ABOUT
THE SAFETY OF EPHEDRA

There has been much confusion and alarm in recent times
about the risks and possible dangers of products containing
ephedra. Many of the reports of problems with ephedra are
incomplete, inaccurate, or irrelevant. Clearly, some of this
misinformation and alarm has been and continues to be generated by the FDA itself, and much of it has been the product
of irresponsible journalism, whether in the form of newspa-
per stories or television specials. There is, however, a wealth
of documentation about the long-term safety record of products containing ephedra and considerable scientific evidence
of such safety for most individuals.

The Council for Responsible Nutrition (CRN) released
a report on December 20, 2000 that concluded ephedra is
safe when ingested as a dietary ingredient in a dietary sup-

plement and where the ephedrine content does not exceed 30 mg per serving and 90 mg per day. The report was prepared by Cantox Health Sciences International (Cantox), an independent scientific consulting firm. The report was based on a review of 19 previously conducted clinical trials, including research recently completed by scientists at hospitals associated with Harvard and Columbia Universities.

Cantox found no evidence of adverse events in its review of the 19 studies, but did acknowledge that certain people, such as those with heart disease, diabetes, and many other ailments, should not consume ephedra. That conclusion is consistent with the standard warning recommended by the dietary supplement oriented trade associations, which is included on the label of most ephedra-containing products. The 30 mg/90 mg levels found to be safe by Cantox are far greater than the 8 mg per serving and 24 mg per day limitations, now withdrawn, that the FDA proposed in 1997.

Dr. Joseph A. Levitt, Director of the FDA's Center for Food Safety and Applied Nutrition (CFSAN), stated that the FDA would review Cantox's report and all science-based information submitted to the Agency regarding the safety of dietary supplements containing ephedra alkaloids. He also stated that the FDA will not make any final decision regarding the fate of the pending regulation of ephedrine alkaloid-containing dietary supplements before the end of calendar year 2001.

The FDA became very concerned about the safety of ephedra-containing products in the mid-1990s following a flurry of activity in Texas about the supplement, Nature's Nutrition Formula One. The Texas Department of Health (TDH) had received a handful of consumer injury complaints from one of that state's Poison Control Centers. The follow-up activity led to investigations by the TDH and the FDA and to numerous civil lawsuits. The FDA held a meeting during October 11–12, 1995 of its Food Advisory Committee; that Committee and outside experts considered the safety of dietary supplements and herbal teas that contain ephedrine alkaloids. The reason given in the announcement for this meeting was:

> Over the past few years FDA has received widespread reports of injuries that may be associated with food products with ingredients such as Ma huang and Chinese ephedra. . . . The committee will hear FDA and outside presentations on the significance and extent of serious adverse events related to these products. The events include chest pain, myocardial infarction, hepatitis, stroke, seizures, psychosis, and death.

Subsequently, the FDA established a reporting "Hot Line," dubbed "MedWatch," for consumers to call and report medical problems with supplement products containing ephedrine alkaloids. MedWatch can be accessed at *www.MedWatch.com*. The result was that the FDA received approximately 900 Adverse Event Reports (AERs), including about 40 deaths, purportedly caused by ephedrine alkaloid-containing products.

These AERs have been exhaustively reviewed by the FDA, consumer groups, and industry-related scientists and lawyers. An industry group of companies that manufacture or distribute products containing ephedrine alkaloids, the Dietary Supplement Safety and Science Coalition (DSSSC), responded to the challenges, conclusions, and diatribe of TDH and the FDA by hiring well-known, experienced toxicologists to review each AER. Their general conclusion was that over 85 percent were unreliable and flawed in their methodology, information gathering, lack of completeness, lack of consistency, analysis, and logic.

Another indication of a flawed basis was the substance of the reports about deaths reported in the AERs. One was caused by gunshot wounds; one was due to hypothermia; and, in one case, a person with huge amounts of alcohol in his blood was going 90 mph the wrong way on a one-way street.

These AERs were the basis for the FDA's Proposed Rule. The Government Accounting Office (GAD) critiqued the information-gathering of the FDA (its Medwatch method) and its analysis of the AERs and the resulting Proposed Rule. Largely because of the GAO Report on the AERs, the FDA withdrew major sections of the Proposed Rule (see below).

FDA's Proposed Rule—June 1997—and Industry Response to the Proposed Rule in Comments

The FDA proposed a new rule about ephedra alkaloid-containing products in June of 1997. It would have limited serving sizes (this is a food term as contrasted with "dosages," a drug term) to 8 mg of ephedrine with a 24 mg daily maximum for no more than 7 days. Regulation 62 Fed. Reg. 30678 (June 4, 1997) was proposed to be added to the Code of Federal Regulations at 21 C.F.R. §111.100. The Proposed Rule contains several other provisions, including a mandatory warning that ingesting more than the recommended serving of ephedra may cause death, and a prohibition of ephedrine-caffeine combinations. When the comment period on this Proposed Rule expired on December 2, 1997, the agency had received hundreds of comments and objections from consumers and industry participants.

The FDA sent a letter to Congress on February 25, 2000 in which it set forth its priorities regarding the regulation of dietary supplement products that contain ephedrine. Among other things, the FDA made announcements in the *Federal Register* that concerned two specific components of its previously-issued year 2000 plan.

First, the FDA announced that the Adverse Event Reports it received after the publication of the 1997 Proposed Rule is available to the public. It also made public, on March 31, 2000, its analysis of these reports pursuant to the Freedom of Information Act.

Second, on June 4, 1997, the FDA issued a Proposed Rule with respect to dietary supplements containing ephedrine alkaloids. The FDA withdrew several provisions of this Proposed Rule on Apil 3, 2000. Below is a table that (1) identifies each provision of the Proposed Rule, as it was published on June 4, 1997, and (2) states whether the FDA has withdrawn or retained the provison.

Provision of the June 4, 1997 Proposed Rule	Status of the Provision
Dietary supplements shall not contain more than 8 mg of ephedrine alkaloids in a single serving.	Withdrawn
Dietary supplements shall not recommend or suggest conditions of use that would result in the intake of 8 mg or more of ephedrine alkaloids within a 6-hour period, or a total	Withdrawn

daily intake of 24 mg or more of ephedrine alkaloids.

The FDA will use a "high performance liquid chromatography method" to determine the level of ephedrine alkaloids that are present in a dietary supplement.	Withdrawn
The label of a dietary supplement that contains ephedrine alkaloids shall state "Do not use this product for more than 7 days."	Withdrawn
No ingredient, or ingredient that contains a substance, that has a known stimulant effect may be included in a dietary supplement that contains ephedrine alkaloids.	Retained
No dietary supplement that contains ephedrine alkaloids may, expressly or implicity, purport to be or be represented as for use for long-term effects, such as weight loss or body building.	Withdrawn
The label or labeling for a dietary supplement that contains ephedrine alkaloids that, expressly or implicitly, purports or is represented to be for short-term effects, such as increased energy, shall state "Taking more than the recommended serving may cause heart attack, stroke, seizure, or death." Specific requirements regarding the placement and type size of this statement apply.	Withdrawn
The labeling of any dietary supplement that contains ephedrine alkaloids shall prominently and conspicuously bear the following warning:	Retained

"**WARNING:** If you are pregnant or nursing, or if you have heart disease, diabetes, high blood pressure, depression or other psychiatric condition, glaucoma, difficulty in urinating, prostate enlargement, or seizure disorder, consult a health care provider before using this product. Do not use if you are using monoamine oxidase inhibitors (MAOI) or for 2 weeks after stopping a MAOI drug; certain drugs for depression, psychiatric or emotional conditions; drugs for Parkinson's Disease; methyldopa; or any product containing ephedrine, pseudoephedrine, or phenylpropanolamine (ingredients found in allergy, asthma, cough/could, and weight-control products). Stop use and call a health care professional immediately if dizziness, severe headache, rapid and/or irregular heartbeat, chest pain, shortness of breath, nausea, noticeable changes in behavior, or loss of consciousness occur. Do not exceed the recommended serving.

Several states have promulgated regulations or enacted statutes that address the sale, labeling, and/or advertising of dietary supplements containing ephedrine alkaloids in various forms, such as extracts of the ephedra plant and ephedrine hydrochloride (EHCl).

Ohio was among the first states to enact a statute regarding ephedrine-containing dietary supplements. The Texas Department of Health, promulgated a very comprehensive set of regulations regarding ephedrine-containing dietary supplements in 1999. Several other states regulate these dietary supplements with varying degrees of restrictiveness.

Ohio Law

The Ohio legislature enacted a statute that permits the sale of ephedrine-containing dietary supplements under certain conditions. This law has been used as a model by other states when considering similar legislature. The Ohio statute includes these provisions: First, the product may not contain EHCl or other hydrochloride or sulfate salts of ephedrine alkaloids. Second, Ohio law imposes a maximum of 25 mg of ephedrine alkaloids per serving. Third, the product label must prominently disclose the following information:

1. the amount in milligrams of ephedrine alkaloids in a serving or dosage unit;

2. the amount of the food product or dietary supplement that constitutes a serving or dosage unit;

3. the maximum recommended dosage of ephedrine for a healthy adult human is the lesser of 100 milligrams in a 24-hour period for not more than twelve weeks or the maximum recommended dosage *or* period of use provided in applicable regulations adopted by the United States Food and Drug administration; and

4. that improper use of the product may be hazardous to a person's health.

Fourth, ephedrine-containing dietary supplements may not be sold or given to persons under the age of 18, except when dispensed by a pharmacist or physician. Fifth, advertising and promotional claims may not represent that an ephedrine-containing dietary supplement causes euphoria, a "buzz" or "high," or an altered mental state; heightens sexual performance; or because it contains ephedrine alkaloids, increases muscle mass. Claims related to increased muscle mass can be made if the claims relate to other ingredients in the product.

TEXAS LAW

The TDH regulations, which were the result of multiyear hearings and other input, address three issues surrounding ephedrine-containing dietary supplements: (1) sale and distribution, (2) product labels, and (3) advertising and promotional literature.

TDH regulations prohibit the sale of dietary supplements that contain EHCl or other forms of ephedrine that TDH considers to be "chemically synthesized ephedrine group alkaloids"; only ephedrine extracted from the ephedra plant is permitted. Additionally, each batch of the finished product sold in Texas must be analyzed to ensure that it contains the total amount of ephedrine alkaloids listed on the product's label.

TDH regulations require the labels for ephedrine-containing dietary supplements to contain the following information: (1) the amount, in milligrams, of ephedrine alkaloids and other ingredients, such as caffeine, that are known to have a stimulant effect; (2) standardized nomenclature for the active ephedrine ingredient, such as "ephedrine" or "pseudoephedrine" in place of or in addition to botanical names, such as ephedra *Ma huang*; and (3) labels must include a warning, displayed on the information panel, in distinct contrast to other printing, in at least 1/16-inch type, and must include, at minimum, the following information:

(a) **WARNING:** Not for use by individuals under the age of 18. Do not use if pregnant or nursing. Consult a physician or licensed health care professional before using this product if you have, or have a family history of, heart disease, thyroid disease, diabetes, high blood pressure, recurrent headaches, depression or other psychiatric condition, glaucoma, difficulty in urinating, prostate enlargement, or seizure disorder, if you are using a MAO inhibitor, or any other dietary supplement, prescription drug, or over-the-counter drug containing ephedrine, pseudoephedrine, or phenylpropanolamine (ingredients found in certain allergy, asthma, cough/cold and weight-control products).

(b) Exceeding recommended serving may cause serious adverse health effects including heart attacks and stroke.

(c) Discontinue use and call physician or licensed health care professional immediately if you experience rapid heartbeat, dizziness, severe headache, shortness of breath, or similar symptoms.

(d) Consuming caffeine with this product may cause serious adverse health effects.

(e) Sale to persons 17 or younger is prohibited.

Beginning on September 1, 2001 labels must include a toll-free number for consumers to report adverse effects that may be a result of consuming ephedrine-containing dietary supplements to the FDA's MedWatch product reporting program.

TDH regulations also place numerous restrictions on the advertising of ephedrine-containing dietary supplements. All advertising and promotional literature must be approved by the manufacturer and submitted to TDH. Advertising claims may not suggest the use of the product for euphoria, as a legal alternative to an illicit drug, or to diagnose, treat, cure, or prevent a disease. Additionally, direct marketers are partially responsible for ensuring that their distributors, franchisees, and independent contractors do not make representations regarding the medical effects of ephedrine-containing dietary supplements.

REGULATION BY OTHER STATES

Hawaii enacted legislation in 1999 that permits the sale of dietary supplements that contain extracts from the ephedra plant. However, this legislation prohibits the sale of dietary supplements that contain EHCL.

In Idaho, the sale of ephedrine-containing dietary supplements, whether the product contains an extract of the ephedra plant, EHCL, or some other form of ephedrine, is effectively prohibited due to the Idaho Board of Pharmacy's interpretation of a regulation known as Exemption 02 of Rule 158 ("Exemption 02"). Exemption 02 exempts certain products from Rule 158's requirement that products containing ephedrine alkaloids may only be dispensed pursuant to a prescription. Exemption 02 could be interpreted to exempt dietary supplements that contain limited amounts of ephedrine alkaloids for the prescription requirement. However, the Idaho Board of Pharmacy has issued an official interpretation of Rule 158, which provides that the listing of ephedrine as an ingredient, including the term "ephedrine alkaloids," anywhere on a product label removes the product from Rule 158's exemption.

This interpretation contradicts the requirements of Texas, Ohio, and many other states, which require the amount of ephedrine alkaloids present in a product to be disclosed on the product's label. Since it is impossible to concurrently comply with Idaho law and the law of numerous states, the sale of ephedrine-containing dietary supplements without a prescription in Idaho is effectively prohibited.

State authorities in Nebraska have interpreted the ephedrine laws of their state in a manner similar to that in which the Idaho Board of Pharmacy interprets Rule 158. Any non-OTC drug product containing ephedrine alkaloids, whether from an extract of the ephedra plant, EHCl, or some other form of ephedrine, may only be dispensed pursuant to a prescription.

A bill that was introduced in the California State Assembly in early 2000 would have imposed requirements and restrictions nearly identical to the TDH ephedrine regulations. That bill, however, was never enacted.

Numerous other states, including Indiana, Kansas, Arizona, and Michigan, have bills pending that address ephedrine, primarily in the context of controlling its use in the manufacture of methamphetamine. It is possible that these bills, if enacted, would affect the sale of ephedrine-containing dietary supplements depending on how they are interpreted and applied.

Idaho is an example of a state whose law regarding ephedrine is aimed primarily at controlling the manufacture of methamphetamine, but the application of which effectively prohibits the sale of ephedrine-containing dietary supplements.

THE GAO REPORT CRITICIZING THE FDA'S AERS—JULY 1999

On July 2, 1999, the General Accounting Office (GAO) issued a report entitled "Dietary Supplements: Uncertainties in Analyses Underlying FDA's Proposed Rule on Ephedrine

Alkaloids." The main GAO findings that are presented in this report are the following:

1. The FDA did not establish a causal link between the ingestion of ephedrine alkaloids and the occurrence of adverse events for either the FDA's proposed dosing level of 8 mg per serving or duration of use of 7 days.

2. The FDA's proposed restriction to an amount of 8 mg per serving was based solely on information associated with only 13 Averse Event Reports (AERs) out of 864 AERs that the agency had received on dietary supplements containing ephedrine alkaloids. An example of an adverse event is an increase in heart rate. A "serious" adverse event would be a stroke.

    A. The number of AERs (i.e., 13) used to support the dosing regimen was small; and

    B. The quality of these AERs was questionable.

3. The FDA did not perform a causal analysis to determine whether the reported events in these 13 AERs were, in fact, caused by the ingestion of dietary supplements containing ephedrine alkaloids.

4. Numerous problems with the 13 AERs were found which raised questions about the causal relationship between ingestion of the implicated product and the adverse events that occurred.

    A. In 3 AERs, physician reports were included that stated the cause of the adverse event was not related to a dietary supplement; and

    B. Three individuals reported having experienced similar problems prior to using the dietary supplement.

5. Uncertainties exist in the FDA's analysis of the relationship between duration of use of dietary supplements containing ephedrine alkaloids and the occurrence of adverse events.

6. The FDA did not present scientific evidence, which specifically pointed to an increase in adverse events after 7 days of normal use of dietary supplements containing ephedrine alkaloids.

  A. Instead, the FDA relied on scientific information that outlined problems with extended use in terms of months and years; and

  B. The use of AERs to describe a pattern of response across time is questionable because the FDA indicated 10 to 73 percent of the reported adverse events might not be related to the consumption of dietary supplements containing ephedrine alkaloids.

7. The AERs, as a whole, lacked data or had inconsistent information (e.g., any preexisting conditions, the amount of product used, how often it was used, or how long it was used), which was relevant to the FDA's analysis and its decision to promulgate the proposed rule.

  A. Sixty-two percent of the GAO's random sample of the 864 AERs did not contain medical records, which are important for determining potential underlying conditions that might have caused the adverse event; and

  B. In the same sample, cases existed in which the amount of product consumed or the duration for which it was consumed was listed differently in multiple locations in the same AER.

Based on these findings, the GAO recommended that before proceeding to final rulemaking, the FDA needed to provide stronger evidence on the relationship between the intake of dietary supplements containing ephedrine alkaloids and the occurrence of adverse reactions, in order to support the serving size and duration of use limits in the FDA's proposed ephedra rule. The FDA concurred with the GAO's recommendation and has already begun to accumulate additional information to determine the degree of support for the requirements in the Proposed Rule. Accordingly, the underlying "science" for the FDA's ephedra rule should be given no weight until more scientifically significant results are obtained.

RECENT DEVELOPMENTS

Dr. Christine A. Haller and Dr. Neal L. Benowitz, medical doctors at the University of California, San Francisco, at the request of the FDA, conducted an independent review of 140 adverse event reports submitted to the FDA via its MedWatch program. The purpose of the review was twofold: (1) to assess causation; and (2) to assess the level of risk the use of supplements containing ephedra alkaloids pose to consumers.

The result was a very controversial article entitled "Adverse Cardiovascular and Central Nervous System Events Associated with Dietary Supplements Containing Ephedra Alkaloids," published in the *New England Journal of Medicine*, with a publication date of December 21, 2000, but released on November 7, 2000. Dr. Haller is a postdoctoral researcher in the laboratory of the senior author, Dr. Benowitz, who is a professor of medicine, psychiatry, and biopharmaceutical sciences at the UCSF-affiliated San Francisco General Hospital Medical Center. Their report included a finding that

Thirty-one percent of cases were considered to be definitely or probably related to the use of supplements containing ephedra alkaloids, and 31 percent were deemed to be possibly related. Among the adverse events that were deemed definitely, probably, or possibly related to the use of supplements containing ephedra alkaloids, 47 percent involved cardiovascular symptoms and 18 percent involved the central nervous system. Hypertension was the single most frequent adverse effect (17 reports), followed by palpitations, tachycardia, or both (13); stroke (10); and seizures (7).

Ten events resulted in death, and 13 events produced permanent disability, representing 26 percent of the definite, probable, and possible cases." Their conclusion was: "The use of dietary supplements that contain ephedra alkaloids may pose a health risk to some persons. These findings indicate the need for a better understanding of individual susceptibility to the adverse effects of such dietary supplements.

Scientists and trade association groups' such as the American Herbal Products Association' voiced and published their critiques and rebuttals. Dr. Theodore Farber sent a Letter to the Editor of *Prevention* magazine (Feb. 2001 issue) condemning the magazine's portrayal of the Haller and Benowitz article as "the truth." Dr. Farber wrote: "As an expert in toxicology and pharmacology, I can assure you that ephedra is indeed safe for weight loss when used as directed. Your conclusion that it is unsafe is based on a scientifically flawed analysis that the FDA used in 1997 to publish limits

on ephedra products. The flaws in the analysis were confirmed in a report issued by the General Accounting Office in
August 1999."

How Ephedra Products Are Covered in the Popular Press, and Its Effects on U.S. Regulation

Pressure from the media is resulting in increased action by
the FDA with respect to the dietary supplement industry.
News and magazine articles in the popular press often state,
erroneously, that the dietary supplement industry is unregulated, or that "there are no laws governing dietary supplements"; and these pieces almost always emphasize the
negative aspects of the industry. Such stories appear in *USA
Today* and *Time* magazine, as well as in reputable and well-
respected newspapers like *The New York Times* and the
Washington Post.

Ephedra commands headlines because of the popularity
of diet products, and, we believe, because of the continuing
misreporting of the AERs collected and analyzed by the
FDA. Here is the beginning of an Associated Press article,
which is fairly typical: "The 38-year-old California man
gulped his usual two capsules of the herbal supplement
ephedra with a cup of coffee, then went on his daily jog. Later
that morning, he dropped dead from cardiac arrest."

Less dramatic and more objective than the print media
is coverage appearing on the Internet. For example, a piece on
the WebMD Web site of August, 7, 2000 was entitled "Is
Ephedra Safe?" with the subtitle "Panel of Experts Say,
Generally, Yes; Still, Controversy to Continue." In this bal-
anced article, rather than alarmist misinformation, is the fol-

lowing: "Drawing their conclusions from a review of about 1,200 side effects reported to the FDA, the seven-member panel said Monday that conservative estimates show that there is no greater risk of heart-related side effects occurring in ephedra users than in the population at large." Finally, one lawyer is quoted as suggesting that the FDA would spend its resources more wisely in monitoring and pursuing the "street drugs" containing ephedra (like Herbal Ecstasy), rather than legitimate dietary supplement manufacturers.

More recently, an article in the February 12, 2001 issue of *U.S. News and World Report*, entitled "The Risks of Natural Cures," scrutinized the labels, safety, and efficacy of dietary supplements, and also cited lack of government regulation. An article entitled "Americans Favor Regulation of Dietary Supplements," which appeared on the Yahoo! News Web site *dailynews.yahoo.com*, on March 28, 2001, states that dietary supplements are "largely unregulated in the U.S." Additionally, the article states that an analysis of six national surveys shows that 80 percent of Americans favor giving the FDA more control over dietary supplement manufacturers. One organization dedicated to providing unbiased facts is the Ephedra Education Council, an industry group that provides information from both government and industry on its Web site *www.ephedrafacts.com*.

THE ROLE OF CONGRESS

Meanwhile, Congress is also keeping a watchful eye over dietary supplements and diet products in particular, in part because the FDA has yet to issue GMPs for dietary supplements. At a March 20, 2001 hearing before the United States House of Representatives Committee on Government

Reform, which specifically addressed the regulation of dietary supplements, Joseph A. Levitt, Director of CFSAN, addressed the issue of safety, with respect to dietary supplements generally, and with respect to ephedrine-containing dietary supplements. Mr. Levitt informed the committee that a high priority of CFSAN is to identify important safety issues and to initiate enforcement actions against unsafe dietary supplement products and ingredients. He also stated that CFSAN is continuing to review the scientific evidence and AERs related to dietary supplements that contain ephedrine-alkaloids, as well as public comments related to the August 2000 public meeting of the FDA on the issue of dietary supplements that contain ephedrine-alkaloids.

THE INSPECTOR GENERAL ON THE FDA

The Office the Inspector General (IG) of the United States Depart-ment of Health and Human Services publicly released a report in late April of 2001 that summarizes its evaluation of the FDA's Adverse Event Reporting system for dietary supplements (AERs). The purpose of the IG's evaluation was to determine how well the FDA's AERs functions as a consumer protection tool.

The IG made several findings in its evaluation of the FDA's AERs. First, the FDA's AERs detects less than 1 percent of all adverse events. Second, the FDA cannot properly analyze most of the adverse event reports that it does receive because the reports often lack necessary information about the medical records, product, manufacturer, and consumer that are at issue. Third, the FDA has a limited amount of clinical information about dietary supplements due to the fact that the vast majority of dietary supplements may be marketed without pre-market safety studies. Fourth, the FDA rarely takes safety actions that concern dietary supplements due to these deficiencies in the AERs.

The IG made four recommendations based these findings:

(A) The FDA can facilitate greater detection of adverse events by: (1) requiring dietary supplement manufacturers to report serious adverse events that are reported to them by their consumers; (2) establishing contracts with Poison Control Centers (PCCs) to obtain adverse event reports that these PCCs receive; (3) make health professionals and consumers aware that the AERs are available to them to report illnesses or injuries that they believe may be associated with a dietary supplement.

(B) The FDA can obtain more information that is necessary to effectively evaluate the adverse event reports that it does receive by: (1) educating health professionals about the importance of including medical information in the adverse event reports; (2) requiring dietary supplement manufacturers to register themselves and their products with the FDA; (3) notifying manufacturers when the FDA receives a serious adverse event report; (4) emphasizing to health professionals and consumers the importance of identifying the alleged injured party so that the FDA may follow-up with that party if necessary; and (5) developing a better computer database to track and analyze the adverse event reports that the FDA receives.

(C) The FDA can better control the safety of dietary supplements by: (1) issuing a guidance document that outlines the type of safety information that manufacturers should include in their pre-market notifications for new dietary ingredients; (2) exploring the possibility of a monograph system for dietary supplements that would contain safety information on particular ingredients; (3) collaborating with the National Institutes of Health in setting a research agenda addressing safety issues; (4) assisting the United States Pharmacopoeia in standardizing dietary supplement ingredients, particularly botanicals; and (5) expediting the development and implementation of good manufacturing practice (GMPs) that will allow the FDA to be assured of the precise contents of each batch of supplements that is manufactured in the United States.

(D) The FDA should disclose more information to the public about adverse events associated with dietary supplements. This could include providing information on the FDA Web site that would allow consumers to evaluate for themselves whether a particular adverse event was actually related to a specific product or ingredient.

Appendix A to that report is entitled "FDA's Experiences in Overseeing Ephedrine Alkaloids." In that five-page appendix, the Inspector General used ephedrine alkaloid-containing products to illustrate the FDA's inability to adequately confirm and analyze adverse event reports.

Appendix A

Programs at a Glance

The following charts offer a quick and easy reference for each profile. Remember, you can substitute natural supplements for prescription medications of the same type, and you can mix supplements and medications together, so long as you **do not mix supplements and medications that do exactly the same thing. For example, do not mix N-Profile supplements with N-Profile prescription drugs.**

Prescription Medications

	Phentermine	Phendimetrazine	Tenuate	Effexor® XR	Prozac®	5-HTP (5mg) + Carbidopa (10 mg)	Wellbutrin
N-Profile (hunger, ADD, insatiability, cravings, exhaustion, depression)	37.5 mg at 11 A.M. (on an empty stomach)	35 mg twice a day (if needed) OR	75 mg at 4 P.M (if needed)	—	—	—	—
S-Profile (sweet cravings, compulsive eating, food obsession, bingeing, depression, anxiety/panic, phobias)	30 mg at 11 A.M.	—	—	37.5 mg with food OR	10 mg a day OR	Twice a day	—
D-Profile (depression, addictions, sexual dysfunction, cravings for fatty or salty food)	30 mg at 11 A.M.	—	—	37.5 mg with food	—	—	150 mg every 12 hours
C-Profile (medications alone don't work)	30 mg at 11 A.M.	—	—	37.5 mg with food	—	—	150 mg every 12 hours plus low carb diet

For maintenance, take meds only on Monday, Wednesday, and Friday, **or** take them every day and cut the dosage in half.

Natural Supplements

	Ma Huang or Country Mallow (ephedra)	Green Tea Extract (caffeine)	Tyrosine	5-HTP (sublingual)	5-HTP (supplement)	SAMe (L-methionine & S-adenosyl)	phenylalanine
N-Profile (hunger, ADD, insatiability, cravings, exhaustion, depression)	From 6 to 24 mg at 11 A.M. and 4 P.M.	200 mg twice a day	250 to 1000 mg twice a day	—	—	—	—
S-Profile (sweet cravings, compulsive eating, food obsession, bingeing, depression, anxiety/panic, phobias)	From 6 to 24 mg at 11 A.M. and 4 P.M.	200 mg twice a day	—	As needed to curb cravings (with ephedra or phentermine) OR	50–100 mg three times a day 20 minutes before meals	—	—
D-Profile (depression, addictions, sexual dysfunction, cravings for fatty or salty food)	From 6 to 24 mg at 11 A.M. and 4 P.M.	200 mg twice a day	—	As needed to curb cravings (with ephedra or phentermine) OR	50–100 mg three times a day 20 minutes before meals	1–3 grams a day with a B6 supplement OR	200 mg a day
C-Profile (supplements alone don't work)	From 6 to 24 mg at 11 A.M. and 4 P.M.	200 mg twice a day	—	As needed to curb cravings (with ephedra or phentermine) OR	50–100 mg three times a day 20 minutes before meals	1–3 grams a day with a B6 supplement OR	200 mg a day plus Low Carb Diet

For maintenance, take supplements only on Monday, Wednesday, and Friday, **or** take them every day and cut the dosage in half.

Appendix B

Manufacturers of Medications and Supplements

MEDICATIONS

Effexor . . . Wyeth Ayerst Pharmaceuticals
P.O. Box 8299
Philadelphia, PA 19101
Phone: 610-688-4400
Web page: www.wyeth.com

Prozac . . . . Eli Lilly and Company
Lilly Corporate Center
Indianapolis, IN 46285
Phone: 800-545-5979
Web page: www.dista.com

Celexa . . . . Forest Pharmaceuticals
13600 Shoreline Drive
St. Louis, MO 63045
Phone: 800-678-1605
Web page: www.forestpharm.com

Serzone . . . Bristol-Myers Squibb
Worldwide Medicines Group World Headquarters
Route 206 and Provinceline Road
Princeton, NJ 08543
Phone: 800-489-1845
Web page: www.bristolmyerssquib.com

Wellbutrin . . GlaxoSmithKline
5 Moore Drive
P.O. Box 13398
Research Triangle Park, NC 27709
Phone: 888-825-5249
Web page: www.gsk.com

SUPPLEMENTS

All . . . . . . The Vitamin Shoppe
Catalog Phone: 800-223-1216
Retail Phone: 800-361-1155
Web page: www.vitaminshoppe.com
Comment: Good prices and large selection

All . . . . . . Puritan's Pride
Phone: 800-645-1030
Web page: www.puritan.com
*Comment: Good quality and excellent sales
department*

Appendix *C*

Weight Loss Doctors Near You

Alabama . . . . . JAN McBARRON, M.D.
Georgia Bariatrics
1625 East University Drive
Suite 114
Auburn, AL 36830
Tel: 334/826-0888
Fax: 334/836-0208

Alaska. . . . . . . ALEX BASKOUS, M.D., M.P.H.
Weight Loss Management Specialist
Alaska Regional Hospital
2841 DeBarr Road, Suite 22
Anchorage, AK 99508
Tel: 907/279-4953
Fax: 907/278-4141

Arizona . . . . . . MITCHELL EDELSTEIN, D.O.
2101 N. Country Club Road, #105
Tucson, AZ 85716
Tel: 520/326-2228
Fax: 520/326-5823

P. SCOTT RICKE, M.D.
5700 E. Pima Street
Suite D
Tucson, AZ 85712
Tel: 520/323-8083
Fax: 520/323-0865

DONALD S. ROBERTSON, M.D., MSC
Medical Director
Southwest Bariatric Nutrition Center
7331 E. Osborn Drive
Scottsdale, AZ 85251-6450
Tel: 480/949-5566
Fax: 480/946-0293

Arkansas . . . . . RICHARD S. CLARK, M.D.
208 Shoppingay
West Memphis, AR 72301
Tel: 870/733-1280
Fax: 870/732-2129

California . . . . . ED J. HENDRICKS, M.D.
1700 Alhambra
Sacramento, CA 95816
Tel: 916/736-1999

2310 Professional Drive
Roseville, CA 95661
Tel: 916/773-1191

Colorado . . . . . . W. L. ASHER, M.D., F.A.S.B.P.
7325 S. Pierce Street, Suite 102
Littleton, CO 80128
Tel: 303/972-9138
Fax: 303/933-1876

SCOTT BARCLAY, M.D.
Arapahoe Medical Weight Control
14000 Arapahoe Road, #300
Englewood, CO 80112
Tel: 303/632-3656
Fax: 303/632-3626

Connecticut . . . . RALPH J. LaGUARDIA, M.D.
Renaissance Spa
10 Higgens Highway, Suite 4
Mansfield Center, CT 06250-1437
Tel: 860/456-7101

Delaware . . . . . ZEINA JEHA, M.D., M.P.H.
Cedar Tree Medical and Urgent Care
Center
RR 01, Box 360, Longneck Road
Millsboro, DE 19966
Tel: 302/945-9730
Fax: 302/945-9732

CALVIN THOMAS WILSON II, M.D.
Gynecologist, Bariatrician, Personal Trainer
Wilson Gynecology and Fitness
737 South Queen Street
Dover, DE 19904
Tel: 302/734-9200
Fax: 302/735-8851

**District of
Columbia** . . . . . HERMAN DANIELS, M.D., M.S.
Bariatrics Weight Loss, Inc.
1712 Eye Street N.W., Suite 1004
Washington, DC 20006
Tel: 202/296-5284
Fax: 202/466-4515

RONALD M. JOHNSON, M.D., F.A.S.B.P.
1800 Eye Street N.W., Suite 401
Washington, DC 20006
Tel: 202/737-6868
Fax: 703/836-6678

Florida . . . . . . LEONARD HAIMES, M.D., F.A.S.B.P.
Haimes Centre Clinic—Anti-Aging
Institute
7300 N. Federal Highway, #100
Boca Raton, FL 33487
Tel: 561/995-8484
Fax: 561/995-7773

JEFFREY D. KAMLET, M.D.
300 Arthur Godfrey Road, Suite 200
Miami Beach, FL 33140
Tel: 305/604-9595
Fax: 305/604-9591
E-mail: kamletmd@bellsouth.net

DAISY MEREY, M.D., Ph.D., F.A.A.F.P.
Medical and Bariatric Clinic
200 Butler Street, Suite 201
West Palm Beach, FL 33407
Tel: 561/659-6756
Fax: 561/659-6817

Georgia . . . . . . JAMES T. ALLEY, M.D.
Georgia Center for Anti-Aging Medicine
2518 Riverside Drive
Macon, GA 31204
Tel: 912/745-3727
Fax: 912/745-1974

DARRYL S. GROSS, M.D.
Medical Weight Loss Institute
2280 Salem Road, Suite 102
Conyers, GA 30013
Tel: 770/860-8860
Fax: 770/860-8890

JAN McBARRON, M.D.
Georgia Bariatrics
2904 Macon Road
Columbus, GA 31906
Tel: 706/322-4073
Fax: 706/322-4786

DAVID M. NELSON, M.D.
Square One Medical Weight Control
463 Johnny Mercer Boulevard, Suite B-8
Savannah, GA 31410
Tel: 912/897-3500
Fax: 912/897-9972

Illinois . . . . SHELDON S. GREENBERG, M.D.
University of Chicago Hospital
4646 N. Marine Drive, 7 N.W.
Chicago, IL 60640
Tel: 773/564-5313
Fax: 773/275-6690

Indiana . . . . . . GLENN SHERMAN, D.O.
Spencer County Medical Center
559 Main Street
Rockport, IN 47635
Tel: 812/649-2271
Fax: 812/649-4867

Kansas . . . . . . RICK TAGUE, M.D., M.P.H.
Center for Nutrition
6730 S.W. 29th Street
Topeka, KS 66614
Tel: 785/273-4443
Fax: 785/228-9892

Kentucky . . . . . JAMES A. CUNNINGHAM, M.D.
Mount Vernon Weight Loss Center
P.O. Box 216
25 Richmond Street
Mount Vernon, KY 40456
Tel: 606/256-4102
Fax: 606/256-4093

Louisiana . . . . . TOMAS BIRRIEL, M.D.
P.O. Box 3433
912 Marguerite Street
Morgan City, LA 70381
Tel: 504/384-7173
Fax: 504/384-7057

Michigan . . . . . JEROME W. COOPER, D.O.
Medical Weight Loss Clinics
6008 Pebble Lane Court
West Bloomfield, MI 48322
Tel: 248/353-8446
Fax: 248/855-9767

KATHLEEN M. KLEINERT, D.O.
28803 W. 8 Mile Road, Suite 102
Livonia, MI 48152
Tel: 248/477-2600
Fax: 248/477-5781

Minnesota . . . . . DONALD WILLARD HERRICK, M.D.
Herrick Medical Weight Management
P.O. Box 16169
Minneapolis, MN 55416-0169
Tel: 612/473-5082
Fax: 612/473-9125

Missouri . . . . . . BRENDA WELLS, M.D.
6409 E. U.S. Highway 60
Rogersville, MO 65742
Tel: 417/833-1100
Fax: 417/753-7790

Montana . . . . . KATHLEEN T. BASKETT, M.D.
2835 Fort Missoula Road
Suite 102
Missoula, MT 59804
Tel: 406/542-3687
Fax: 406/327-4475

Nebraska . . . . . JEFFREY PASSER, M.D., F.A.C.P.
9300 Underwood Avenue, Suite 250
Omaha, NE 68114
Tel: 402/398-1200
Fax: 402/398-9119

Nevada . . . . . . CAROLYN PRICE, M.D.
222 S. Rainbow Boulevard
Suite 115
Las Vegas, NV 89145
Tel: 702/255-4325
Fax: 702/255-7660

New Jersey . . . . BYONG K. PARK, M.D.
United Medical
612 Rutherford Avenue
Lyndhurst, NJ 07071
Tel: 201/460-0063
Fax: 201/460-1684

New York . . . . . KALPAMA DESAI, M.D.
A Better You Medical Center
1 Paris Road
New Hartford, NY 13413
Tel: 315/734-1001
Fax: 315/798-9743

North Carolina . . GEORGE BARTELS, M.D., F.A.A.F.P.
204 Ashville Avenue, #50
Cary, NC 27511
Tel: 919/233-6644
Fax: 919/233-8344

MARTA M. KALINSKI, M.D.
Kalinski Health Center, P.A.
3315 Springbank Lane
Suite 304
Charlotte, NC 28226
Tel: 704/295-1252
Fax: 704/295-1255

Ohio . . . . PORTIA VERA CRUZ-CANOS, M.D.
Ironton Bariatric Clinic
1920 S. 9th Street
Ironton, OH 45638
Tel: 740/532-0220
Fax: 740/532-5088

KEVIN D. HUFFMAN, D.O.
18660 Bagley Road
Phase 1, #207
Cleveland, OH 44130-3480
Tel: 440/239-0540
Fax: 440/239-0545

PAUL WEHRUM, SR., D.O., F.A.C.O.F.P.
Severence Medical Arts
5 Severance Circle, Room 604
Cleveland Heights, OH 44118
Tel: 216/291-3223
Fax: 216/291-5642

Oklahoma . . . . . MICHAEL STEELMAN, M.D., F.A.S.B.P.
13301 N. Meridian, Bldg. 400
Oklahoma City, OK 73120
Tel: 405/755-4600
Fax: 405/755-4837

Oregon . . . . . . S. KATHLEEN HIRTZ, M.D.
1800 Centennial Boulevard
Suite 6
Springfield, OR 97477
Tel: 541/726-1865
Fax: 541/726-2179

Pennsylvania . . . HARVEY S. KLEINBERG, D.O.
Healthwise Medical Weight Loss Centers
6518-22 Lebanon Avenue
Philadelphia, PA 19151
Tel: 215/473-7577
Fax: 215/473-3102

SHEONATH P. SRIVASTAVA, M.D.,
F.A.C.G.
Healthy Living Medical Center Inc.
222 Broad Street
Johnstown, PA 15906
Tel: 814/535-3568
Fax: 814/539-9606

Rhode Island . . . AUGUSTUS F. MARSELLA, D.O.
Steven Medical Building
712 Oaklawn Avenue
Cranston, RI 02920
Tel: 401/942-0050
Fax: 401/942-1534

South Carolina . . Charles T. GOODSON, M.D.
Bariatric Medical and Surgical Clinic
2311 Sunset Boulevard
West Columbia, SC 29169
Tel: 803/796-3820
Fax: 803/796-3804

ROBERT M. JOHNSON, M.D.
P.O. Box 1375
Gaffney, SC 29342
Tel: 864/489-1446
Fax: 864/489-4909

A. RANDALL MOSS, M.D.
P.O. Box 1375
Gaffney, SC 29342
Tel: 864/489-1446
Fax: 864/489-4909

MILTON D. SARLIN, M.D.
Sarlin Wellness Way
353 E. Blackstock Road
Spartanburg, SC 29301
Tel: 864/574-7774
Fax: 864/574-9797

South Dakota . . . E. W. FILLER, M.D.
Brookings Medical Clinic
400 Twenty-second Avenue
Brookings, SD 57006
Tel: 605/692-6236
Fax: 605/697-6939

Tennessee . . . . . MICHAEL TALBOT, M.D.
DoctorsCare Advanced Medicine
2908 Poston Avenue
Nashville, TN 37203
Tel: 615/369-5555
Fax: 615/369-5559

Texas . . . . G. R. ALBERTSON, D.O.
Weigh of Life
405 S. Main
Monahans, TX 79756
Tel: 915/943-9477
Fax: 915/689-2529

DOLLY P. DOCTOR, M.D.
2114 W. Tennessee
Midland, TX 79701
Tel: 915/686-9999
Fax: 915/685-1700

C. RICHARD MABRAY, M.D.
Mabray Clinic, LLC
303 E. Airline, Suite 5
Victoria, TX 77901
Tel: 361/574-9697
Fax: 361/574-9244

Utah . . . . DAVID B. JACK, M.D., F.A.A.F.P.
9720 S. 1300 E., Suite W100
Sandy, UT 84094
Tel: 801/576-8855
Fax: 801/576-9800

MICHAEL TWEDE, M.D.
324 10th Avenue, Suite 218
Salt Lake City, UT 84103
Tel: 801/576-2366
Fax: 801/576-2369

Vermont . . . . . . MARK J. BUCKSBAUM, M.D.
Center for Integrative Medicine
69 Allen Street, Suite 9
Rutland, VT 06701
Tel: 802/747-7730
Fax: 802/773-1609

Virginia . . . . . . LISA HARRIS, M.D.
The Chase Wellness Center
4660 D Haygood Road
Virginia Beach, VA 23455
Tel: 757/460-4300
Fax: 757/464-3427

Washington . . . . VERN S. CHEREWATENKO, M.D., M.Ed.
Health Max, Inc.
4033 Talbot Road S., Suite 570
Renton, WA 98055
Tel: 206/362-1111
Fax: 425/254-1111

West Virginia . . . DOUGLAS E. McKENNEY, M.D.
Beckley Bariatric Clinic
1838 Harper Road
Beckley, WV 25801
Tel: 304/252-4154
Fax: 304/256-0821

E.O. RUBIO, M.D.
Beckley Bariatric Clinic
1838 Harper Road
Beckley, WV 25801
Tel: 304/252-4154
Fax: 304/256-0821

Canada . . . . . . E. C. SMART-ABBEY, M.D.
5900 No. 3 Road, Suite 415
Richmond, British Columbia
V7C 5A7
Tel: 604/244-9200
Fax: 604/244-9277

Index

E

Eating disorders, 144
Effexor XR, 55–56
  dosage, 55
  phentermine combined with,
    55–56
  phentermine and Wellbutrin com-
    bined with, 66
  side effects, 56
Elderly persons, 130–131
  exercise for, 117, 131
  medication dosage, 131
Emotions, and body weight, 12, 143
Energy level
  and dopamine imbalance, 62
  medical treatment, 66
  natural treatment, 46, 48–49
  and norepinephrine imbalance,
    38
Environment, and body weight, 8,
    19, 141–142
Ephedra, 44–48
  contraindications, 47–48, 157
  country mallow form, 47
  dosage, 44–45
  drug interactions, 47–48, 172
  DSHEA regulation, 159, 162–164
  effectiveness of, 46–47
  ephedra/caffeine (EC), 46–48
  FDA issue with, 45–46, 158–172,
    164–172
  historical view, 159–162
  mechanism of action, 46–47
  side effects, 47
  state regulations, 159–164
  stimulant effects, prevention of,
    145
Ephedrine, and norepinephrine
    release, 46–47
Epigallo catechin gallate, 48
Epinephrine imbalance, and over-
    weight, 21
Essential fatty acids (EFAs), 84–85
  dosage, 85
  food sources, 84

Estrogen, and weight gain, 147
Evans, Gary, 79–80
Evening primrose oil, 85
Exercise, 115–123
  aerobic exercise, 119–120, 122
  for children, 130
  and eating, 123
  and everyday routines, 118–119
  general guidelines, 121
  health benefits, 116
  motivation for, 116–118
  and muscle weight, 123
  for older persons, 117, 131
  plus dieting, effects of, 120–122
  psychological benefits, 115–116
  resistance training, 120
  varying workouts, 122
  for weight-maintenance, 100–101

F

Farber, Dr. Theodore, 181
Fat cells, 127
Fat genes, and cancer, 18
Fat-to-muscle ratio, 123
Fat-storage, and brain, 17–18
Fatty foods
  controlled eating of, 151
  cravings for, 64
Fenfluramine. *See* Phen-Fen
Fiber-rich diets, ineffectiveness of,
    82
Fiber supplement, for constipation,
    41
Fibromyalgia, natural treatment of,
    58, 59
Fight or flight, 38
Flatt, Jean-Pierre, 71
Flax oil, 85
Folic acid
  birth defects prevention, 3
  daily dosage, 104, 139
Food addiction, 13–14
Food choices. *See* Healthful nutrition

213

P

Panic attacks
  and serotonin imbalance, 53–54
  signs of, 54
Paxil
  for obsessive-compulsive disorder
    (OCD), 15
  and weight gain, 54, 152
Phen-Fen, 21–26
  commercial names, 25–26
  effectiveness of, 20–22
  mechanism of action, 21–23
  phentermine, safety of, 26
  side effects, 24–28
  studies of, 20–22
Phentermine, 40–43
  contraindications, 42
  dosage, 42
  drug interactions, 41
  effectiveness of, 40–41
  mechanism of action, 21, 39–40
  rate of weight loss, 40–41
  safety of, 26, 40
  side effects, 41–42
  SSRIs combined with, 55–56
  stimulant effects, prevention of,
    145, 153
  for teenagers, 129
  tolerance to, 42–43
  tyrosine combined with, 49
  Wellbutrin and Effexor combined
    with, 66
Phenylalinine, 67
  dosage, 67
  food sources of, 67
  precautions, 67
Phobias, and serotonin imbalance, 54
Phosphodiesterase, and norepinephrine release, 48
Pima Indians, and obesity, 7
Pindolol, 145, 152, 153
PMS (pre-menstrual syndrome), and
  serotonin, 147
Pondimin. *See* Phen-Fen
Pregnancy, overweight in, 3–4

Primary pulmonary hypertension
  (PPH), and Phen-Fen, 25
Prochnow, James R., 155
Propanolol, and weight gain, 152
Prostate cancer, 3
Protein foods, recommended foods,
  112
Protein shakes, and C-profile diet, 74
Prozac
  dosage, 56
  for obsessive-compulsive disorder
    (OCD), 15
  phentermine combined with, 56
  for seasonal affective disorder
    (SAD), 147
  and weight gain, 152
Pycnogenol, daily dosage, 139

R

Redux. *See* Phen-Fen
Refined foods, avoiding, 113
Resistance training
  body-building supplements,
    136–139
  and metabolism, 120
  and muscle increase, 120
  plus aerobic exercise, 122
Restaurant dining, food choices, 111

S

S-profile, 51–59
  case example, 28
  identification of, 32–33, 52–54
  medical treatment, 54–57, 188
  natural treatment, 57–59, 189
Safer Than Phen-Fen (Anchors), 56
Salty foods, cravings for, 64
SAMe (s-adenosyl L-methionine),
  66–67
  actions of, 63
  dosage, 67
  food sources, 66
  precautions, 67

U

Uterine cancer, 3

V

Vegetables, recommendations, 112
Ventromedial region, hypothalamus, 15
Verapamil, and weight gain, 152
Vincent, Dr. David A., 16
Vitamin E, daily dosage, 104, 139
Vitamins
  antioxidants, 138–139
  recommended supplements, 104

W

Walking, as exercise, 119–120, 122
Weight control approaches
  acupuncture, 76
  amphetamines, 77
  aromatherapy, 77–78
  behavior-modification, 148–149
  Chitosan, 82–83
  chromium, 78–82
  Citrimax, 83–84
  of diet doctors, 91–92
  essential fatty acids (EFAs), 84–85
  fiber-rich diets, 82
  herbal remedies, 86
  hypnosis, 85–86
  medications, 21–26
  scams and frauds, 81
  Slim Fast, 87
  Xenical, 86
  See also Hunger Switch approach
Weight gain
  and antidepressants, 54, 152
  induced by medication, 151–152
  muscle weight and exercise, 123
Weight-gain types
  C-profile, 34
  D-profile, 33–34

N-profile, 31–32
S-profile, 32–33
Weight-maintenance, 98–106
  discussing with physician, 102–103
  exercise for, 100–101
  natural treatment, 100
  and stopping medication, 99, 143–144
Weight training. *See* Resistance training
Weintraub, Dr. Michael, 23
Wellbutrin, 64–66
  for dopamine imbalance, 64–66
  dosage, 65
  mechanism of action, 65
  phentermine and Effexor combined with, 66
  precautions, 153
Whole-grain foods, recommendations, 112
Wirtman, Dr. Judith, 22
Wirtman, Dr. Richard, 17
Women
  estrogen pills, 147
  menstruation, 147
  overweight, health effects, 3
  overweight in pregnancy, 3–4

X

Xenical, 86

Z

Zinc, daily dosage, 139
Zoloft, 55
  for obsessive-compulsive disorder (OCD), 15